CW01551610

the walking cure

By the same author

Non-fiction

Windswept: Why Women Walk

52 Ways to Walk: The Surprising Science of Walking for Wellness and Joy, One Week at a Time

Sleepless: Discovering the Power of the Night Self

The Age-Well Project (with Susan Saunders)

Fiction

The Joyce Girl

Frieda: The Original Lady Chatterley

The Language of Food

ANNABEL STREETS

the walking cure

Harness the life-changing power of
landscape to heal, energise and inspire

TONIC

LONDON • OXFORD • NEW YORK • NEW DELHI • SYDNEY

BLOOMSBURY TONIC
Bloomsbury Publishing Plc
50 Bedford Square, London, WC1B 3DP, UK
Bloomsbury Publishing Ireland Limited,
29 Earlsfort Terrace, Dublin 2, Ireland

BLOOMSBURY, BLOOMSBURY TONIC and the Tonic logo are trademarks of
Bloomsbury Publishing Plc

First published in Great Britain 2025

A catalogue record for this book is available from the British Library

ISBN: HB: 978-1-5266-7632-0; eBook: 978-1-5266-7633-7; ePDF: 978-1-5266-7635-1

2 4 6 8 10 9 7 5 3 1

Commissioning editor: Rowan Yapp
Project editor: Faye Robinson
Design by Clare Baggaley

Printed and bound in Great Britain by Clays Ltd, Elcograf S.p.A.

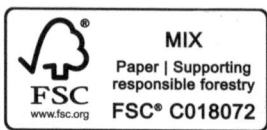

MIX
Paper | Supporting
responsible forestry
FSC
www.fsc.org
FSC® C018072

To find out more about our authors and books visit
www.bloomsbury.com and sign up for our newsletters

For product safety related questions
contact productsafety@bloomsbury.com

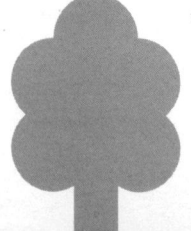

*To Matthew, Imogen, Bryony, Saskia
and Hugo, who walk beside me, always*

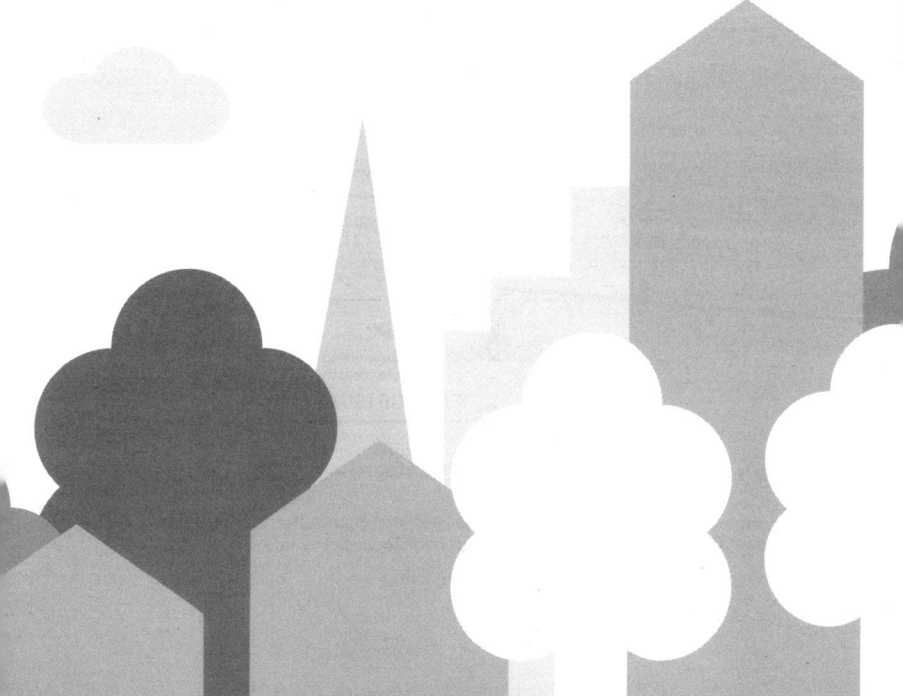

contents

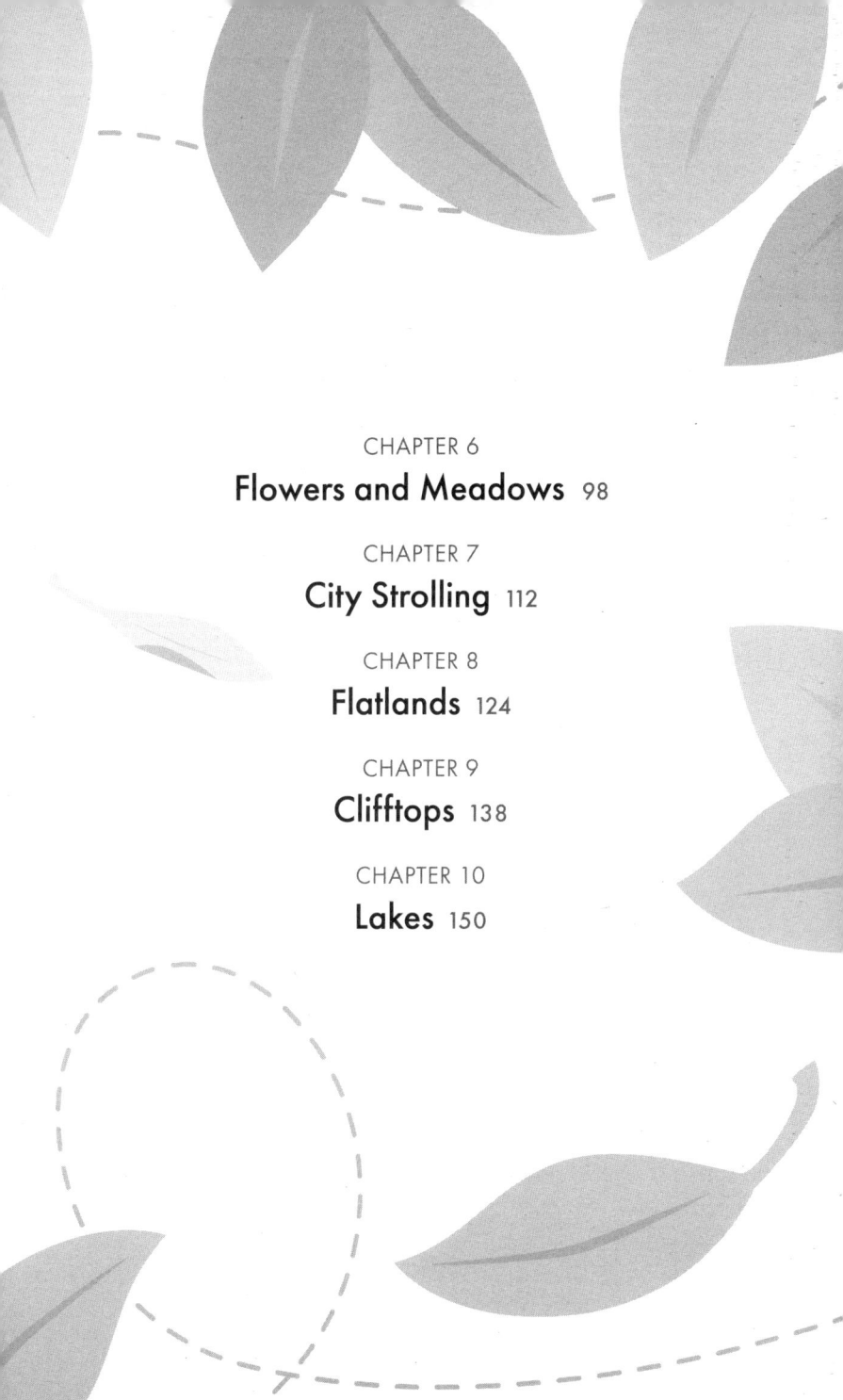

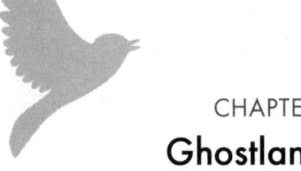

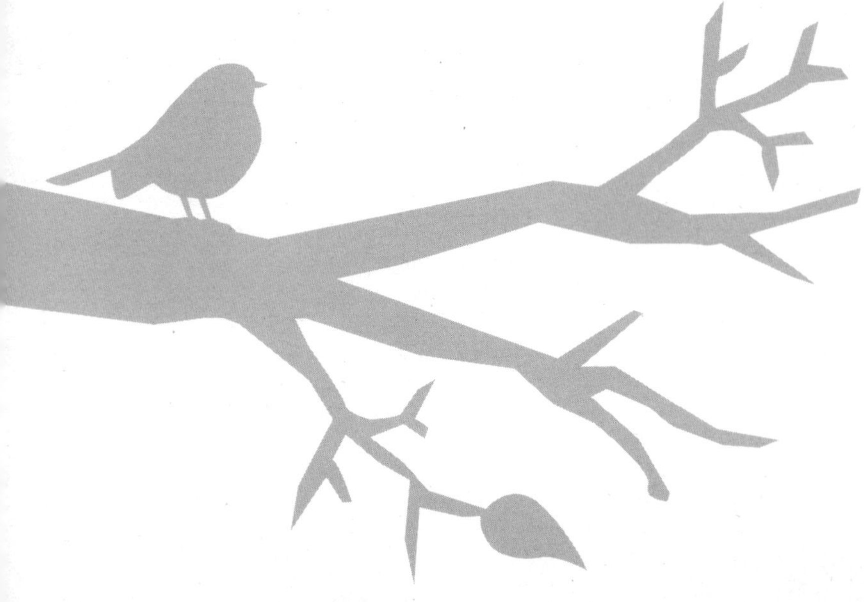

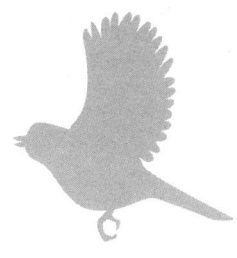

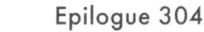

Author's Note

'Health is greatly affected by landscape . . . our mental and physical health depends and relies on it.'

LAURA MENATTI AND ANTONIO CASADO DA ROCHA, 'LANDSCAPE AND HEALTH'[1]

Why do some landscapes call to us at certain times of our life? Why do we sometimes wake up longing for the sea, or craving the fizzing streets of a city? And why do different places make us feel so . . . different?

The Walking Cure uses anecdotal and empirical evidence to examine the interaction between place, body and mind, the mysterious dialogue we have with the earth and the air – and its implications for our wellbeing. It is not intended to dictate *where* we should walk but to illuminate the often muffled longings of our walking self.

Modern life makes it difficult to decipher the call of place. Lost amid the cacophony and comfort of our pixellated age, we can feel utterly disconnected and too bogged down in daily life, too reluctant to step out of our quotidian spaces, to give extended thought to *where* we walk. Listening to our body has never been more challenging. Many of us must relearn the subtle notes of place and space. In order to register the quickened heartbeat and altered emotions – however fleeting, however light-fingered – that come as we move from terrain to terrain, we must plunge back into our skin and bone, we must learn to hear the softest of whispers from the furthest corners of our brains and bodies. We must also learn to quieten our own voice so that we can hear what our landscapes have to say. Sometimes a little bit of knowledge can help us do this.

Introduction

'Sensitivity is the only
answer for understanding
a landscape.'

SARAH MARQUIS, *WILD BY NATURE*

Where do you like to walk? Do you ever find yourself pining for a place, longing for a particular landscape? I do. In the past, I have craved desert, forest, ocean, mountains and city streets. I have yearned for rivers, cemeteries, starlit fields. Not to look at on a screen, but to walk through. At times the call was so consuming I had no choice but to leave my desk and deadlines, find the nearest available location I was hankering for – and walk it.

Later I understood: when my life was overwhelmingly busy and my mind frazzled from too many decisions and too much responsibility, I longed for the uncluttered space of deserts or plains. When things came tumbling down in a deluge of confusion, I needed the airy perspective bestowed by mountains. When I lost confidence, I yearned for the steadfastness of a river. When I felt unmoored by sadness, I wanted the reassuring clasp of trees and woodland. When I felt mired in self-pity, I needed the gratitude prompted by headstones in a cemetery. And when I was bored and restless, only the exuberance of a city would suffice.

I often returned from my walks feeling changed: some routes eased my mind while others challenged it. Some places seemed to intensify my emotions, while others calmed me. It struck me that *where* I walked might be influencing my mood, shaping my thoughts and emotions in the subtlest of ways.

Landscapes speak to us differently at different times, reflecting our moods and thoughts, acting as catalysts while we process complicated feelings, prompting new insights into the workings of our own minds, even spurring imaginative solutions to nagging problems or challenging how we see the world. When a place seems to echo our emotions, we are nudged into acknowledging and accepting them, rather than judging or evading them.[1] Landscapes also allow us to encounter aspects of ourselves that we otherwise repress, suppress or do not give ready expression to. They can be outlets for some of our deepest yearnings – to be free, independent, wild.

The writer and psychologist Dr Sharon Blackie believes that places call to us when we most need them. Lakes beckon, she says, when we need to go more deeply into ourselves. Mountains call when we need space, and deserts appeal when we need to shed scraps of our past.[2] This notion is echoed by writer and podcaster Sarah Wilson, who walks the coast when she needs to ease emotional pain, and tramps forests when she needs gentleness and forgiveness.[3]

The idea that our health and the landscape are intimately bound up isn't new: the earliest cities of China, Greece and Persia included plenty of greenery and water to aid healing. In Europe, the first hospitals were sited within the cloistered, herbal gardens of convents. At the turn of the twentieth century, the model 'garden city' was thought to improve health and happiness. More recently, psychologists at Sweden's Alnarp Rehabilitation Garden and Denmark's Octovia Health Forest have been investigating the therapeutic traits of specific landscapes on the unsettled, burnt-out brain, asking *how* and *why* they help us heal.

> "Meaningful places
> generate a strong
> emotional response . . .
> impacting us physically
> and psychologically"

In the last ten years or so, a handful of environmental psychologists and neuroscientists have started using technology to understand why places affect us, and how physical location can constrain, guide and shape us. A pioneering paper from the National Trust and the University of Surrey found three brain regions that registered powerful responses to landscape: the left amygdala, the medial prefrontal cortex and the parahippocampal place area. According to Professor Bertram Opitz, who led the study, 'the brain treats meaningful places very differently to both objects and everyday places ... meaningful places generate a strong emotional response ... impacting us physically and psychologically'.[4]

Unfortunately, these studies excluded movement. Instead, participants were asked to look at screen images while their responses were monitored, measured and recorded using technologies like fMRI and EEG.*

But here's the problem: looking at a landscape on a screen doesn't deliver what our bodies long for. When we feel the pull of an ocean, forest or mountain peak, a saturated digital image will rarely suffice. Personally, I need full, mobile immersion. I want to feel the salt spray of sea air on my cheeks, or the tug of mountain wind in my hair. I want to breathe in damp moss, spring sap, the first bluebells. I want to smell the freshly brewed coffee and newly baked bread that signifies a city at dawn. Above all, I want to *move through a place*, to see its grasses and buildings change, to sense shale become dune, or turf become reeds, or pavements become parks. I want to see the light softening as morning becomes afternoon. I want my ears full of birdsong,

---

* Functional magnetic resonance imaging and electroencephalogram, both measuring brain activity.

then rushing streams and the scraping of insect wings, followed by the chiming of church clocks and the banter of a city bar.

"Above all, I want to move through a place"

And while all this is going on, I like to feel the pulling and working of my muscles, the swinging of my arms, the steady stride of my feet. Without which a landscape affects us quite differently, as confirmed by researcher Dr Amy McDonnell, who told me that her lab (at the University of Utah) found people were cognitively different when *immersed* in nature: 'there's something unique about the multi-sensory experience of immersion that can't be replicated by just looking at images'.

Fledgling studies are beginning to bear this out – and to pick apart how different forms of immersion affect us.[5] New research suggests that when we exercise near a beach or river, we feel greater self-esteem and better mood than when we exercise in urban green space, farmland or woodland, for example.[6] Studies indicate that walking alone in a maintained forest yields greater mental wellbeing than walking alone in an unmaintained forest.[7]

Group walks across farmland have been found to lower stress more effectively than those taken in urban environments.[8] And yet city strolls have been found more cognitively invigorating than walks through fields.[9] Meanwhile, people who walk beside the sea sleep for longer than those walking elsewhere. It's also becoming apparent that the wildlife of a landscape deeply affects us, with several new studies correlating psychological wellbeing (and sheer joy) with the diversity of bird, butterfly and plant species in the environment.[10]

As one study put it, 'categorizing environments as "natural versus urban" may gloss over . . . the restorative potential of different physical environments'.

But how do we disentangle landscape from movement? For researchers, this is a conundrum: is it the landscape or the act of walking that so radically affects us? And if it's the walking, how much is influenced by speed, intensity and duration? One team, having noticed that all these variables wreaked havoc with their experiments, pointed out that those who walked at a higher speed reported the best post-walk emotional health and concluded that measuring responses to place without considering movement was a big mistake.[11]

How we move, the direction of our movement, even the timing of it, subtly and biochemically alters us. But so does the landscape through which we walk. It could be the chemical compounds (phytoncides) produced by plant life, or the negative air ions that linger around water – both of which change the air we inhale. It could be the memories evoked by a scent on the breeze, the feelings of wonder as we gaze at an unending ocean or a beautiful building, or the curious sense of companionship we find on a canal towpath. It could be the specific molecules activated by our bodies in response to specific locations. Or it could be the way in which our bodies are nudged into moving differently by the landscape itself, shifting our circulating biochemicals yet again. As the neuroscientist Dr Sarah McKay says, 'Your body, how you move it, and how you interact with your physical surroundings shape how you think, feel, and behave ... even altering the structure and functioning of your brain to improve your mental health, memory and cognition.'[12] All of it stirred up in a heady cocktail of mind-bending chemicals.

When we walk, our body and brain produce a cascade of biochemicals – hormones, neurotransmitters, proteins, metabolites, peptides, lipids and acids – that can dramatically affect our wellbeing. These molecules are so powerfully life-enhancing, scientists call them 'hope molecules'.[13] It's thought these sweeping changes in cellular biochemistry do more than simply resolve the body's increased demand for oxygen and nutrients. They also cleverly disguise the potential muscle fatigue, pain and mental stress that can accompany demanding movement – an evolutionary adaptation that ensured our survival as hunter-gatherers.

"These molecules are so powerfully life-enhancing, scientists call them 'hope molecules'"

Perhaps the most critical biochemicals are pain-alleviating endocannabinoids which, once released into the bloodstream, flow smoothly through the blood-brain barrier to the brain, where they blunt any vestiges of anxiety and induce mild sedation and feelings of euphoria. In fact, endocannabinoids do more than this: they also reduce inflammation in the brain, improve memory and help make our brains more plastic.

In the last few years, scientists have uncovered many more 'hope molecules' (also known as exerkines) generated by movement, including:

DOPAMINE: A neurotransmitter (and hormone) involved in pleasure, reward and motivation which appears to be released as we exercise.[14] Dopamine also moderates activity in the brain region that governs fear (the amygdala), making us less anxious.

SEROTONIN: A neurotransmitter (and hormone) that makes us cheerful, energetic and alert, and surges in the blood plasma of exercising rodents and humans. Scientists speculate that low-intensity but acute movement (like hiking or hill walking) is the most effective means of releasing serotonin.[15]

NOREPINEPHRINE/NORADRENALINE: A neurotransmitter boosted by exercise, and thought to manage and modulate other neurotransmitters responsible for our stress response. The more norepinephrine we have, the better we can manage our inner turmoil.[16]

LACTATE: Once considered a waste product that caused sore muscles, lactate is now a potential preventive agent for brain diseases like Alzheimer's and Parkinson's.[17] Lactate also appears to reduce anxiety and increase resilience to stress.[18] Moreover, lactate triggers production of another compound called histone lactylation, thought to play a role in countering diverse conditions, including infection and cancer.[19]

PLATELET FACTOR FOUR (PF4): A protein released after exercise by the tiny blood cells that prevent clotting. New studies have found that PF4 can rejuvenate old brains and boost young brains, 'leading to a brain with less inflammation, more plasticity and ... more cognition', explained Dr Saul Villeda, who helped discover the astonishing potential of PF4.[20]

KYNURENINE: Raised levels of kynurenine, a neurotoxic metabolite, have been found in depressed and frail people, and those with broken or fractured bones. Biologists think that inflammation prompts the body to make more kynurenine, which then triggers the formation of other damaging molecules. Intriguing new research suggests that kynurenine (and its toxic by-products) can be converted to beneficial kynurenic acid during extended periods of movement, with uplifting effects on our mood.[21]

IRISIN: A hormone secreted by skeletal muscle during and after movement, irisin has been linked to improved cognition as well as better heart health, improved metabolism, weight loss and the relief of various symptoms of depression. More recently, irisin has been found to clear the toxic amyloid plaque found in the brains of those with Alzheimer's disease.

BRAIN-DERIVED NEUROTROPHIC FACTOR (BDNF): Commonly known as Miracle-Gro for the brain, BDNF enables nerve fibres in the brain to grow, a process known as neurogenesis. Brisk walking stimulates BDNF – which, in addition to improving cognition, also blunts feelings of depression and anxiety. Some researchers think exerkines work by promoting production of BDNF.

Other hope molecules currently under investigation include cathepsin B, glycosylposphatidylinositol-specific phospholipase D1, oxytocin (see Chapter 11, 'Ghostlands'), osteocalcin, β-hydroxybutyrate, insulin-like growth factor 1 (IGF-1), apelin, and fibroblast growth factor 21 (FGF21). Little wonder, then, that hundreds of reports have found a pulse-raising walk can help numerous disorders of the mind, including depression, anxiety, post-traumatic stress, bipolar and psychosis, while also boosting self-esteem, self-belief, resilience, and feelings of pride, competency and achievement.[22] As Murray Stein, professor of psychiatry and clinical research at the University of California, told the *Washington Post*, movement 'should be prescribed for virtually anything that ails humankind'.[23]

Why does movement have such remarkable effects on our minds? Evolutionary biologists think it was once a survival mechanism – when we ran from danger, our brain had to be as competently efficient as our body. We needed to recognise our location, recall places of refuge, rapidly determine whether to climb a tree, change direction, pick up a rock, slow down or speed up. Effective escape has always required as much brain as brawn, as much intellect as speed. To reward us for our efforts, these chemicals also made us *feel* good, ensuring that we endured and survived, that we never gave up hope.

Interestingly, being awash in hope molecules may also prime us to be more receptive to *where* we are. We may smell and taste more acutely, hear with greater clarity, think more cogently and – thanks to our ebbing introspection – be more open to the magnificence and majesty of the landscape.[24] We benefit physiologically too, because when we run from danger, our entire body has to work as a single, powerful machine, signalling effortlessly between skeleton, liver, muscle, adipose tissue, gut and multiple brain regions. Exerkines ensure this 'cross-talk' happens.

But here's the problem (again): most studies have been done on treadmills in laboratories. The full panoply of benefits that come from walking through a landscape have rarely been tested, measured or scrutinised.

Thanks to new technologies like functional near-infrared spectroscopy (fNIRS), which enable our brains to be examined while on the move, this too is changing – and with intriguing results. In 2022, a group of Korean researchers analysed the growing pile of shinrin-yoku, or 'forest-bathing' studies, and noticed something curious: the higher the forest altitude, the greater the reduction in depression and anxiety. Was it the woodland or the altitude that was having such a dramatic effect, they wondered. Altitude seems to play a larger part in the therapeutic nature of forests than has been accorded, they wrote, adding that 'natural settings do not provide the same uniform health benefits'.[25] Later, when members of the same team investigated further, they found (surprise, surprise) that it wasn't forest *bathing* but forest *walking* that had 'the most consistent positive health effects'.[26]

Weather offers another confounding factor. Studies have found that still water – known for its calming effects – is more emotionally restorative on cloudy days, while open, exposed areas are more physiologically rejuvenating on bright, clear days.[27] Meanwhile, more and more studies are suggesting that air quality plays a significant role – with dirty air consistently wiping out the physical and mental wellbeing bestowed by a landscape. Reports from Denmark and the USA have linked air pollution with depression, anxiety, bipolar disorder, psychosis and suicide. Researchers think air pollutants might be inflaming the brain, causing it to malfunction – another reason to choose our route with care.

The *noise* of traffic can be almost as detrimental, as made clear in a 2023 study carried out in Hong Kong: the researchers expected residents to have 'noise immunity' but were shocked to find that 'residential traffic noise was associated with probable depression and poorer mental wellbeing'.[28]

Studies of ambient temperature reveal that the heat or cold of a place also affects us, with chilling intimations for a globally (and excessively) warmed planet. Equally important (and overlooked in most studies, sadly) are feelings of safety. When we feel perilously unsafe, no amount of beauty, birdsong, breeze or circulating hope molecules can render a landscape healing, therapeutic or even enjoyable.

Most of us are now very familiar with the gifts of so-called 'green' (nature) and 'blue' (water) space. And yet many walking locations – excluded from the original lexicon of therapeutic landscapes – appear to have oddly curative effects, from cemeteries to city squares and standing stones. In this book I examine both the more obvious landscapes, but also the unexpectedly rejuvenating – any of which can kindle a mysterious, intimate fusion of mind, muscle, earth and air.

I hope *The Walking Cure* inspires you to listen closely to your body and your soul, to return to the places you love but also to seek out new and unfamiliar landscapes. As Sharon Blackie says, 'there are times when you need to retreat to the wilderness

. . . [and] times when you need the subtle flow of a river, the song of a waterfall and the deep slow presence of trees'.[29]

To which I'll add: There are times for city parks with their sturdy benches and cool ice creams. There are times when we long for strangeness and obscurity, or for a glistering dome of stars and planets. There are times when we must walk amid the warm press of our fellow humans and times when we want nothing more than an endlessly empty road. There are times when we need the soft sink of sand beneath the soles of our feet, and there are times when we want the solid certainty of a city pavement.

Listen carefully: only you know what you need.

notes

Explore multiple landscapes: when Swiss researchers investigated the emotional and psychological wellbeing of walkers, they found that the more varied locations people strolled, the better they felt.[30] This may be because the exerkines we produce can change according to altitude, temperature, air quality, the effort with which we walk (and so on). Or it may be a result of our brain's innate love of novelty.

Equally, don't worry if you're continually pulled back to the same place. Psychologists have found favourite places serve 'as tools for emotional regulation and self-regulation'. Repeated encounters provide layers of memories which, in turn, deepens and enriches our relationship with our 'chosen place'. Environmental psychologists speculate that having, and visiting, a special, easy-to-reach place helps us transform negative thoughts and feelings into positive ones.[31]

Dr McDonnell thinks of our preferences as *landscape compatibility*, saying different places 'may be differentially restorative to different individuals'. For many of us, our 'happy place' is the landscape of our childhood. Studies show that children with wonderful memories of time spent in pine forests are more likely to find them uplifting.[32]

Equally, there will be occasions when we need landscapes with which we have no emotional connection. These diverse, unknown places can prompt a broader spectrum of emotions: a 2023 Spanish study concluded that 'diversity of landscape' often leads to 'diversity of emotions', which, in turn, resulted in a greater sense of connection to the land.[33]

How long should we walk? According to one study, twenty minutes was sufficient to reduce depression in older people.[34] But as its author told me, 'the more the better'.

Some studies have found that our movement changes according to the landscape (more slowly by water, for example). Pay attention to your own gait and speed as you move from terrain to terrain – do you speed up, slow down, move differently?

Studies suggest that for urban dwellers, 120 minutes in nature each week is all it takes to reap the benefits of green space, either taken as a single two-hour walk or as two hour-long walks.[35] Either way, find time to go somewhere green: studies have found that walking in nature (compared to urban walking) reduces rumination. Urban walking, however, can make us feel more energised.

Blood pressure is affected by *where* we are: cold, altitude, noise and air pollutants can all cause spikes in blood pressure – another example of how sensitive the body is to place and space. Choose with care.

Our microbiome can also be altered by the landscape, thanks to the bacteria we inhale (or absorb via the skin). Trees, plants, water and soil produce beneficial bacteria that adds to the diversity of our own microbiota, with subsequent effects for our mental and physical health.[36] Breathe deeply, stroke tree bark, poke around in moss, soil and seawater.

Endocannabinoids can be amplified by altitude and singing.[37] Follow the example of the von Trapp family – sing as you hike mountains!

Scientists now think we absorb nutrients in the air we breathe: in 2024, two Australian researchers coined the term *aeronutrients* to cover airborne bioactive molecules produced by the landscape. Little wonder that a breath of fresh air makes us feel so good.[38]

Forests and Woodland

A Chemistry Class in
Arboreal Calm

'In the country it seems as if every tree said to me: "Holy! holy!" Who can give complete expression to the ecstasy of the woods! O, the still sweetness of the woods!'

LUDWIG VAN BEETHOVEN

— — — — — — — —

DEFINITION: A large area covered chiefly with trees and undergrowth.

BENEFITS FOR: Loss of faith; craving solitude; insomnia; anger in women; depression in men. In brief, almost everything . . .

I n 1933, the Canadian artist Emily Carr bought herself a clapped-out camper van, named it 'Elephant' and then set off in search of 'deep, quiet woods'. When she found them, she spent days wandering, 'staring, staring, staring' at the trees. She had – finally – discovered an earthly embodiment of God. Inspired, she began to paint the trees and woodlands, which seemed to express 'an attribute of God – power, peace, strength, serenity and joy'. Carr – an introvert with a penchant for the remotest, loneliest corners of forests – befriended the trees, explaining that they 'were better than we humans . . . never in a hurry or behind'.[1] When Carr discovered forests, her search for God and peace finally ended. The 'solemnity, majesty and silence [of the forest] was the Holiest thing I ever felt,' she wrote. God, she added, had grown 'stuffy squeezed into a church'. But in forests and woodlands she found a new God, 'like a great breathing among the trees'.

"Places of creativity, healing and refuge"

The forests became a source of 'great bursts of creative spiritual emotion'[2] for Carr, inspiring some of the greatest forest paintings ever made. A century earlier, Beethoven had made a similar observation, writing to a friend that 'my ideas . . . come unsummoned . . . out in the open air, in the woods while walking'. For Beethoven, trees appeared as sacred things: 'Woods, trees and rocks send back the echo that man desires,' he wrote in an 1815 letter. At the time, Beethoven was tormented and saddened by the progressive loss of his hearing, noting that on his woodland walks, 'my miserable hearing does not bother me'.[3]

Forests, according to Carr and Beethoven, were mysterious portals to transcendence, reminders of life's spiritual dimension. But they were also places of creativity, healing and refuge. So what is it about forests that make them so remarkably curative?

In Japan, following more than two decades of pioneering investigations into shinrin-yoku, forest medicine has become a university subject in its own right – a blend of ecology, biology and functional medicine. Japanese researchers were the first to identify the extraordinary effects of woodland on human health, which include:

- a greater number of natural killer (NK) cells* with anti-cancer properties
- reduced blood pressure, heart rate and circulating stress hormones (namely less urinary adrenaline and noradrenaline and less salivary cortisol)
- increased activity of parasympathetic (rest and digest) nerves and reduced activity of sympathetic (fight or flight) nerves
- boosted immunity
- diminishing feelings of anxiety, depression, anger, fatigue and confusion
- surges in vigour and energy.[4]

More recently, a study of twenty men in their fifties found that four hours of walking in a forest 'significantly increased levels of serotonin' (the oft-called happiness hormone) when compared to walking in a city. The researchers noted that 'forest bathing may have potential preventive effects on depression'.[5] But why are woodlands proving to be such powerfully alchemical places?

Dr Qing Li, the guru of Japanese forest bathing, acknowledges that while the clean air, peace, pleasant aromas and visual

---

* Natural killer cells destroy virally infected cells, and detect and control cancerous cells.

interest of a forest play a part, it is the volatile organic compounds produced by trees to protect themselves that have 'a bigger effect'. It's the phytoncides, he says unequivocally, that increase our anti-cancer NK cells and cut the concentration of adrenaline and cortisol in our blood.[6] 'They improve cardiovascular function, hemodynamic indexes, neuroendocrine indexes, metabolic indexes, immunity and inflammatory indexes, antioxidant indexes, and electrophysiological indexes; [they] significantly enhance people's emotional state, attitude, feelings . . . physical and psychological recovery, and alleviate anxiety and depression.'[7]

Thanks to the work of Dr Qing Li and his team, dozens of forest-based health initiatives have been implemented across East Asia, Europe and North America. Japan now has its own forest-therapy certification system, while Korea has a licence system for trained forest therapists, and at least one German state allows forest therapy to be covered by health insurance.

But not all forest bathing involves walking, which is why we need to pay special attention to the studies that distinguish between walking in forests and 'static' bathing (sitting or meditating, for example). When we untangle some of this data, it becomes clear that walking in a forest ('dynamic forest bathing') has a greater impact on our mental health than remaining static. In one recent study where participants took either hour-long walks or hour-long 'sits', those walking saw significantly greater mood improvements. The researchers concluded that 'dynamic forest bathing shows greater effects on mental health'.[8] It's this magical cocktail of inhaled phytoncides, our in-body walking chemicals, and the sheer sensory magnificence of hundreds of trees that render a forest hike so powerfully regenerative.

Before you rush off to your nearest scrap of woodland, we need to dig a little deeper. Despite the excitement surrounding forest bathing, not all trees and woodlands affect us in the same way. Fascinating new studies reveal that it may only be very old trees and woodlands that alter us, both psychologically and physiologically.

A few years ago, three researchers asked themselves whether all woodlands were capable of producing the same well-known forest-bathing benefits. Fifty-six men and women were asked to walk for half an hour through four different types of forest outside the city of Helsinki: young woodland, old woodland, recreationally designed woodland and mature commercial woodland. At the end of the experiment all participants felt less stressed and more positive, regardless of the type of wood they had walked in. But these gains were most marked after walking through mature and old woodland. The researchers noted that 'it takes decades before a forest provides health benefits', urging forestry personnel to leave woodlands for as long as possible.[9]

"Put simply, large, old trees comfort and calm us"

In the Danish forest laboratory Octovia, an experiment to find the most relaxing type of woodland yielded clear results: 'All participants [were most] affected by the size and appearance of the [old] pines,' wrote the researchers. Put simply, large, old trees comfort and calm us.[10]

It's not only our mood that improves in older woodland. In 2023, Spanish researchers split thirty fibromyalgia patients into two groups, one of whom walked daily in mature woodland while the other walked daily in young woodland (trees less than thirty-five years old). Those walking among old trees reported improvements in pain and insomnia, and greater feelings of good health. But, to the researchers' surprise, these improvements failed to materialise among those walking in younger forests.[11]

What is it about old trees that prompt our bodies to respond so favourably? We know that phytoncides have powerful effects. But here's the thing: mature trees are host to a far greater variety and quantity of these healing molecules than young trees. When we walk through diverse mature trees pumping out diverse phytoncides, we are inevitably exposed to the full healing capabilities of a woodland.

The phytoncide known as a monoterpene (found in conifers, among others) is particularly powerful and appears to calm us. A 2023 experiment in which 500 participants were exposed to monoterpenes from different Italian forests found that participants became more or less anxious according to the levels of terpenes circulating in the air. The more abundant the terpenes, the more relaxed participants felt.[12]

Of course, forests offer more than phytoncides, clean air and glorious smells (for more on mood-enhancing smellscapes go to Chapter 6, 'Flowers and Meadows'). They also gift us closed and secluded spaces, which environmental psychologists often refer to as places of refuge. Here we can be protected from the elements, but we can also feel hidden from other people. More than any other landscape, forests and woodlands offer shelter and solitude. If we see someone coming, we can dive behind tree trunks, clamber into branches, duck beneath weeping boughs, or simply slip further into the forest.

When researchers surveyed students in the grip of various negative moods, they found that the closed and semi-closed landscapes offered by woodlands had particular appeal to those feeling angry and those with 'esteem-related moods'. When we don't wish to be seen by others, or to socialise in any way, when we need to be utterly alone with ourselves, forests offer us sanctuary and refuge.

In the Alnarp Rehabilitation Garden (see Introduction), researchers noticed that those who drifted towards the forest garden (the wildest, most wooded area) commented not only on its serenity and seclusion but its perceived safety. Here, they knew they 'could be alone ... to hide and find a nice sheltered place where one could "see others but not be seen" ... participants told how they could move around without being heard or seen, and hide from the rest of the world'.[13]

"Trees can provide a sense of companionship that mitigates loneliness"

And yet we are never truly alone in a forest. Trees (particularly mature trees) are magnets for wildlife. The insects they host are food for birds, while their limbs provide habitats for moss, fungi and climbing plants. Trees can provide a sense of companionship that mitigates loneliness, giving us, instead, the solitude craved by Emily Carr and enjoyed by Beethoven.

I often feel the mysterious tug of the forest. From nowhere I find myself yearning to walk between trees. In my nearest woodlands the trees are colossal, cathedral-like, their branches forming vaulted, shady walkways. No doubt the phytoncides are working on my cells. But what really strikes me is the rootedness of the vast oaks, the sturdiness of the tall beeches, the strength and heft of the lofty pines. I find them deeply reassuring. I take comfort from knowing that they have been here for centuries, that they will outlive me and my family. That they will be encountered by generations to come. In an uncertain and endlessly changing world, I appreciate their predictable, steadfast presence. They ask nothing of me, and yet give so much – arboreal medicine, reassurance, sounds that uplift, shade in summer, food for thousands of insects and birds, a trunk to hide behind, branches from which to hang wet coats and walking poles, fuel for a fire (should we need one) – and endless fascinating distraction, thanks to the fractal intrigue of their leaves, bark, and the lichens and moss that live on them.

notes

Look for forests with an abundance of ancient trees. Don't be afraid to touch or hug them – grounding studies (see Chapter 2, 'Shorelines') suggest we can benefit from the earth-to-root exchange of electrons that takes place when we touch a tree. Meanwhile, studies of skin microbiota have found that those who handle greenery have enhanced immunity (see Chapter 6, 'Flowers and Meadows').

Most 'tree therapy' or shinrin-yoku studies are carried out in woodlands that are not only mature but also heavily coniferous. Indeed, evergreen trees are thought to be richer in phytoncides – so seek out forests with a good scattering of mature evergreens.

A few early studies have found a difference in the responses of men and women to forest walks – with men reporting less subsequent depression and fatigue, while women report dramatic dissipation of anger. A 2022 study suggests that (in women but not in men) a forest walk blunted the amygdala, the brain part instrumental in feeling fear and rage. The baffled researchers noted 'that amygdala activity decreased after the walk in nature, but only in women'.[14] Listen carefully to your own body: how does a forest walk make *you* feel?

Some walkers are frightened of forests and yet most forests are perfectly safe. Take a leaf out of Emily Carr's book and treat your fear not as an impediment but as creative fuel.[15] Alternatively, walk with a friend.

Short of time? Studies suggest that the effects of a forest are noticeable within minutes of entering, and rise the longer you spend there, lingering for a further seven days.

Can't sleep? A two-hour afternoon walk in a wood improved the sleep of seventy-one insomniac participants in a 2005 experiment, 'impacting actual sleep time, immobile minutes, self-rated depth of sleep, and sleep quality', wrote the authors.[16]

Try not to plug into music or podcasts: the three sounds that most soothe our churning minds are birdsong, wind and water – all of which are readily found in forests.[17]

In need of spiritual restoration? Danish researchers found that a sheltered environment – but with views out – was the best place for spiritual recovery.[18]

The same Danish researchers also found that environments 'rich in species' were highly effective at countering stress and burnout. Look for large forests with a wide variety of trees, lots of open and closed space, and plenty of water – all of which ensure a greater diversity of flora and fauna.

Avoid dense, dark woodland – when researchers monitored the brains of walkers, they found a raised pulse rate in very dense forests, but signs of relaxation in forests rated as medium-dense.[19]

Numerous studies have confirmed that forest smells – earth, wood, pine needles – are deeply relaxing. Inhale (through your nose) as you walk, or buy a good, scented 'forest' oil and put a few drops, nightly, into a diffuser (see Chapter 6, 'Flowers and Meadows' for more on the sorcery of scented plants).

Levels of phytoncides vary according to time of day and year, peaking in the early afternoon, especially in the summertime but also in the early morning.[20] Other factors affecting the amount of circulating phytoncides include meteorological conditions, altitude, seasons, sunlight exposure and tree species. Studies indicate that the most phytoncide-rich woodlands include a mix of coniferous and broad-leaved trees.

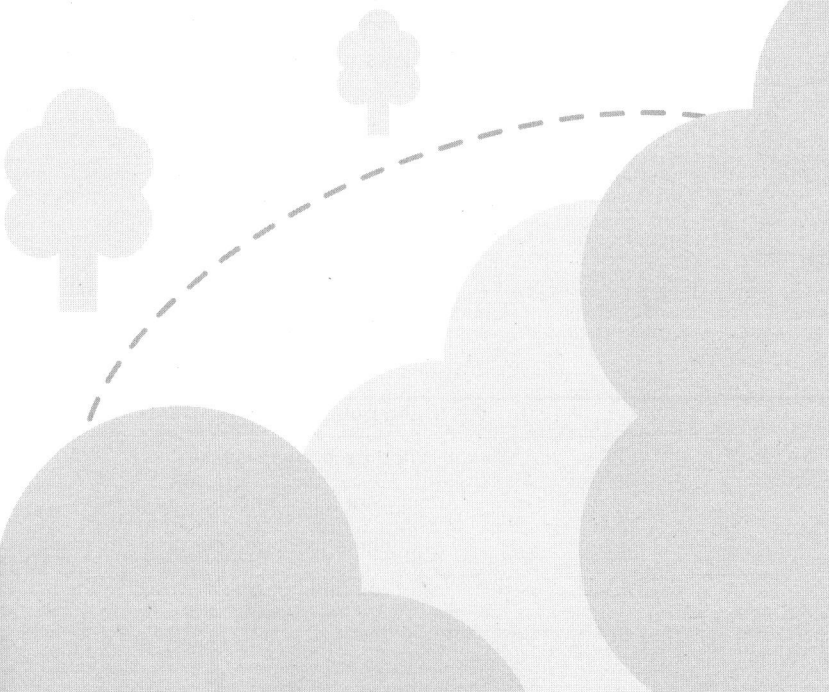

Shorelines

The Surprising Science of Sea, Sand and Shingle

'In front, like an immense window, is the infinite horizon, always the same, yet always new . . . I begin to breathe, to admire, as I stroll along.'

MARIE BASHKIRTSEFF, FROM *MARIE BASHKIRTSEFF: THE JOURNAL OF A YOUNG ARTIST*

— — — — — — — —

DEFINITION: A strip of land covered by sand, shingle or small stones at the edge of a body of water, especially by the sea between high- and low-water marks.

BENEFITS FOR: Accepting or dispersing feelings of grief, loss, sadness. Worry. Cravings for space after long confinements. Sleeplessness.

I n December 2022, Cleo Shaw was bone-tired. Jonathan Shaw's slow descent into dementia had been agony to watch and exhausting to manage. Every muscle in Cleo's body ached. Her brain throbbed in a semi-permanent migraine. And now Jonathan no longer recognised his wife of forty years.

'It was the final straw,' she explained. 'He was alive but not the man I married. I knew we couldn't go on like this but I persevered in a fog of tiredness and despair.'

Eventually Cleo snapped. 'I hadn't left the house for months and I saw the sudden smallness of my world. I realised that I was no longer a very good or happy carer. Something had to change.' She made the most difficult and painful decision of her life: to put Jonathan into a nursing home. 'I was racked with guilt,' she said, 'but then something extraordinary happened. My legs started to twitch, often uncontrollably – not painfully, but as if they wanted to be moving, walking.'

After settling Jonathan into a home, Cleo decided to out-walk the twitching in her restive legs. 'I wanted to say a slow goodbye to the husband I'd once had,' she added. 'I knew the caring wasn't completely over, so I also needed to be repaired and restored. A long walk on my own seemed to be the answer.'

Cleo wasn't sure where to go. But as she studied maps and routes, strange sounds began to mass in her ears. 'At first I thought there was something wrong with my hearing, but then I recognised the sounds – they were softly rolling waves. The ocean seemed to be calling me.'

After hiking a section of the Welsh Coastal Path, Cleo suddenly understood: 'I'd lived with the smell of sickness for years, in a cramped, airless space. I needed sea winds to blow the taint from me, and I needed the huge expanse of ocean to free me from all the uncomfortable emotions I'd lived with for so long. The seashore is a place of letting go and I returned home a different woman.'

"The sea activates all our senses"

According to Dr Catherine Kelly, author of *Blue Spaces: How and Why Water Can Make You Feel Better*, Cleo's experience isn't unusual. When Kelly unexpectedly lost her own mother, she too felt the pull of the ocean: 'I needed to get my head cleared . . . to be blown away by the wind and nature.' For Kelly, a geographer, the tug was 'instinctive and intuitive'. She bought a house on the Irish coast and walked a three-mile beach twice a day. 'It healed me,' she explained.[1]

A few years later, Kelly began researching the remedial power of water. 'The sea activates all our senses, taking our attention away from our thinking brain,' she explains. 'With water we are instantly and effortlessly mindful, which also slows our breath, cutting off the neural path to the amygdala.' Which is to say, we feel less anxious and fearful.

Kelly's ideas are supported by the latest studies which show that the more contact we have with 'blue space', the more restored we feel.[2] And particularly so in coastal landscapes. A recent Japanese study found that 'the beach has a great influence on improving mood and mental health', reflecting numerous earlier studies that have linked time at the coast with greater feelings of satisfaction and significantly less anxiety and depression.[3]

"Coastal air includes miniscule droplets of seawater – rich in iodine, magnesium, calcium and potassium"

Researchers think the reason we feel so good at the beach might be due to inhaling coastal air, which includes miniscule droplets of seawater – rich in iodine, magnesium, calcium and potassium. They suspect that inhaling these minerals could soothe the mucosal lining of our respiratory system, relieving symptoms of asthma and stimulating the immune system to clear waste from our lungs. Indeed, studies of patients with lung disease found that spells of ocean air resulted in less coughing and improved lung function.[4] To boot, Italian researchers noticed that there were far fewer Covid hospitalisations in coastal areas, suggesting that sea air had reduced the hospital burden (by 1,363 cases to be precise!).[5]

And this isn't all. Early studies of sea air have found it contains tiny bioactive molecules derived from ocean-dwelling plants, algae and creatures: bacteria, vitamins, pigments, polyphenolics and phycotoxins.[6] Much as forests and woodlands have their own airscape (see Chapter 1, 'Forests and Woodland'), so does the beach.

Intrigued by the possible therapeutic benefits of these ocean-blown molecules, Belgian researchers exposed human lung-cancer cells to sea air (in petri dishes) and found that the cancer cells subsequently shrunk. They speculated that these bioactive molecules could be contributing to the health effects associated with coastal environments. Pharmaceutical companies are now investigating yessotoxin, a bioactive molecule produced by plankton, which appears to reduce melanoma cells in mice. Excited researchers describe it as having 'important potential . . . as an anti-cancer drug'.[7]

Nor is it just cancer tumours that respond to sea air (in petri dishes – just to be clear). It's possible that inhaling the wide range of biogenic chemicals yielded by sea air could help rid our bodies of the damaged cells that form brain plaques found in Alzheimer's disease. These pioneering studies are still in their infancy, but could they explain why so many reports[8] have found people living near the sea to be in possession of superior physical health? In 2023, scientists published a study spanning fifteen countries confirming, once again, that those living nearest the sea reported better health than those living inland. Luckily for those of us without a beach house, this study also found a role for visits to the coast: seaside visits, it stated, 'have substantial effects on health'.[9]

"Part of the sea's mentally curative effects can be credited to its sheer size"

Marine scientist Michael Moore believes the complex chemical makeup of sea air could ease the effects of inflammation, known to be a causal factor in cardiovascular disease, depression, neurodegeneration and dementias, as well as in many cancers.[10]

As you breathe deeply of the sea air, be sure to look into the horizon. It appears that part of the sea's mentally curative effects can be credited to its sheer size. When researchers in the lake-rich state of Michigan examined the hospital records of people admitted for mood disorders, they were astonished to find that those living closest to the largest lakes appeared to be the least afflicted, concluding that 'only larger water bodies' were genuinely therapeutic.[11]

The more I beach-walked, the more I began to wonder whether something extremely simple might also be contributing to my subsequent (good) mood. After all, the expansive views and sea air could be experienced merely by sitting. I decided that it was the act of walking over stones, shingle and sand – a mode of moving that was slow and physically demanding. Walking on sand requires around 2.7 times more energy expenditure than walking on a solid surface at the same speed.[12] All our lower body muscles, and particularly those at the knee and hip, must work harder as we attempt to stabilise ourselves on shifting sand and stones, making a beach stroll the equivalent of walking up a constant 2 per cent incline, and resulting in significantly increased muscle mass in multiple lower-limb muscles.[13]

In other words, as we walk over shifting dunes, undulating sand and rattling pebbles, our body works at an accelerated rate, flooding our brain with: feel-good, pain-blocking endocannabinoids; anti-inflammatory platelet factor 4 (PF4); vivifying dopamine and noradrenaline; and joy-inducing serotonin and oxytocin (see Introduction and Chapter 11, 'Ghostlands'). Which might explain why a National Trust study found coastal walkers experienced deeper and longer slumber than their inland-walking peers – sleeping for an additional forty-seven minutes.[14]

Meanwhile, the slowed pace gives us ample time to take in the sequinned light, the salt-sharp breeze, the silver sea stretching forever into the horizon. To walk over similarly gruelling surfaces in any other landscape would be dully exhausting. But beside the sea, we are so calmed and distracted, we barely notice.

"Being in direct physical touch with the earth for an hour dramatically lifted the mood of participants"

There's another possible factor in the alchemy of a seaside stroll: walking barefoot. Early studies suggest that taking off our shoes and socks prompts a foot-brain connection with repercussions for our cognition.

In 2016, bemused researchers discovered that barefoot runners had better 'post-run' memory than their shod counterparts, particularly after jogging over poker chips (which we might think of as beach shingle). Something about being shoeless on an uneven, unfamiliar surface appeared to sharpen the memory.[15]

Eight years later, a Korean team of researchers conducted an experiment in which participants (some barefoot and some in trainers) walked for fifty minutes a day over twelve weeks while having their brain waves scanned using EEG.[16]

EEG measures four types of oscillating brain waves (H-beta,

M-beta, SMR and alpha), each of which is associated with a particular state of mind, from deeply focused to calm and relaxed. The barefoot walkers showed very different EEG results, with increased levels of all four brain waves. Walking barefoot seemed to result in a greater sense of relaxation, as well as an enhanced ability to focus, concentrate and remember. Walking without shoes, noted the researchers, can 'activate the enteric nervous system, increase brain blood flow and stimulate the toes ... leading to improved overall cognitive ability.' The foot-brain connection needs more research, but it seems that walking safely barefoot could benefit our brains and our mood, as well as our balance, gait and muscle.

Finally, when we walk barefoot we might experience the benefits of grounding (sometimes called earthing). Proponents of grounding believe that when our skin touches the earth's surface, free electrons are absorbed into our bodies, where they make their way to places of inflammation, triggering a form of healing. Think of it as akin to the way in which we make vitamin D from the sun's energy. Grounding merely involves energy and frequencies from beneath our feet.

For years I was sceptical of grounding. But recent peer-reviewed studies in scientific journals suggest that my scepticism may have been premature. An experiment carried out in 2015 found that being in direct physical touch with the earth for an hour dramatically lifted the mood of participants.[17] A second experiment reported that those who experienced regular grounding had better mood and less fatigue and depression, while tests also revealed improvements in their inflammatory biomarkers, blood viscosity and heart-rate variability.[18]

Researchers are now pondering whether the earth's current, having passed into the body, might moderate our production of cortisol (too much of which can lead to depression, anxiety and insomnia[19]). When stressed rats had their brains scanned after spending time on earthing mats, they had far fewer of the neuropeptides known to trigger stress hormones. The rats were – quite simply – biochemically calmer.[20] Other small studies have found that earthing minimises blood clotting, which helps reduce the risk of cardiovascular disease.[21] We can earth ourselves almost anywhere, but nowhere lends itself to going barefoot better than a sweep of sun-warmed, sea-cooled sand.

notes

The sea can also be enjoyed from cliff tops and promenades, avoiding sand and shingle altogether (see Chapter 9, 'Clifftops').

Dr Lewis Elliott (who has researched the effects of coastal landscapes) says a two-hour beach walk once or twice a week is all it takes to reap rewards.[22]

Coastal areas have higher ultraviolet (UV) levels, giving beach walkers more access to vitamin D – but also to possible sunburn. Cover up and use sunscreen, whatever the weather.

The air near rolling bodies of water contains abundant negative air ions. See Chapter 19, 'Rivers', for more on these remarkable molecules.

Poor toe-grip strength is increasingly linked to falls later in life. Walking barefoot on sand is one of the best ways of building foot and toe muscle, while also conditioning the feet, according to the American Orthopaedic Foot and Ankle Society. So take your shoes off!

Want to experiment with grounding? Studies show that when the soles of the feet are damp and the earth moist, grounding is more effective.[23] So walk on wettish surfaces where possible. Alternatively, opt for earthing shoes, which include a copper button on the sole to conduct electrons from earth to body.

Wondering how long you need to walk the beach barefoot to experience the (possible) effects of earthing? Apparently thirty minutes is all it takes . . .[24]

Dr Kelly thinks the sociability of a beach adds to its therapeutic powers. Make a point of greeting dogs, walkers, fishermen, wild swimmers, anyone at all.

Look for clean, remote beaches: chemical contaminants (including air pollution), harmful or toxic algal blooms and pathogens can be higher in busy beaches and estuaries close to industrial/urban areas. Download a free app like Safer Seas & Rivers Service (from Surfers Against Sewage in the UK) to find clean, sewage-free beaches.

Can't get to the sea? Panic not – other aquatic locations can be almost as therapeutic. Try Chapter 10, 'Lakes'.

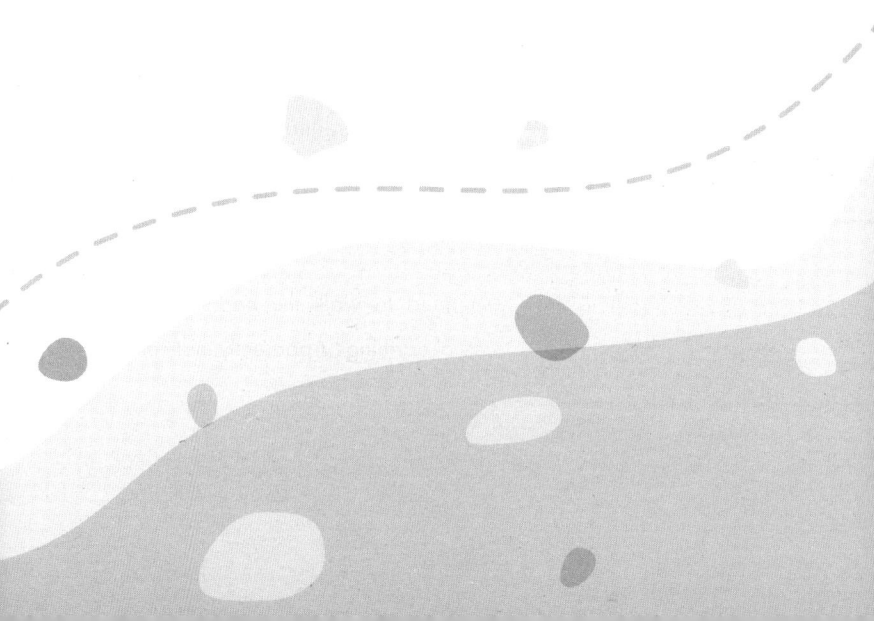

Leafy Lanes and Rural Roads

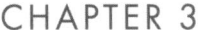

Purpose, People, Pace and
Unexpected Wildlife

'I have always found congenial companionship in English lanes. Their friendly hedges and banks, rich in living things, set up a shelter between me and a hostile world.'

— — — — — — — —

DEFINITION: A narrow country road, often bordered by hedges or ditches

BENEFITS FOR: Wanderlust; purposelessness; aloneness; a compulsion to shed the endless trappings of a consumer lifestyle; a desire to witness the fully man-made landscape, warts and all; forgotten wildlife.

As I researched favourite places to walk, country lanes cropped up repeatedly. When I polled readers of my blog, country lanes made the sixth spot – rather to my surprise. Country lanes felt safe, said respondents ... the homes passed, the dogs barking at gates, the cows peering curiously from behind hedges. 'You can't get lost,' said one respondent. 'No frisky bullocks or biting horses,' said another.

People liked the sense of a clear destination – with either a pub to quench the thirst or a church to explore. Many liked the even, dry terrain. Not only did this smoothed surface enable them to take wheelchairs and pushchairs, and to walk without expensive hiking boots, it also allowed them to pick up – and maintain – a good pace.

Country lanes aren't usually considered a 'landscape'. A century ago, the poet Edward Thomas lamented that 'Much has been written of travel, far less of the road', while reminding his readers that the road was of utmost importance, 'a silent companion, always ready for us, whether it is night or day, wet or fine, whether we are calm or desperate, well or sick'.[1] And yet most walkers will, at some point, find themselves on a lane or a narrow rural road – the pleasure of which will be determined by the volume and speed of traffic. But if you find yourself walking ancient, verdant and quiet lanes, you may have hit the jackpot of landscapes.

"Verges are home to an extraordinary variety of wildlife"

'A lane is beautiful at all times,' wrote Nancy Price in *The Heart of a Vagabond*, her 1955 memoir of road walking. 'Particularly in spring, when the banks are covered with white violets, the hedges bridal with blackthorn blossom and the birds in full song.' Price was writing in the 1950s, and yet road verges are still home to an extraordinary variety of wildlife – 720 different flowers in the UK, which is almost half of all British wildflower species. Verges are also home to a staggering twenty-nine of Britain's fifty-two wild orchid species.[2]

"Many country lanes now form a vital network of wildlife corridors"

Many lanes are flanked by archeologically important banks, ditches and hedgerows, carrying the last remaining seeds of plants that once grew in the surrounding meadows but have been lost as a result of development and industrial farming. These verges and banks provide a vital habitat for insects, spiders, small mammals and birds. Indeed, many country lanes – thought to have existed first as animal tracks – now form a vital network of wildlife corridors.

Nor is this confined to the British Isles. European lanes offer similar possibilities, with a recent study finding that French lanes had more abundant insects living in their verges than anywhere else. In fact, researchers have identified the verges and hedges of France's country lanes as vital hotspots for pollinators.[3]

The 'lush banks' and 'tall thick hedges' of quiet lanes, wrote Price, 'had often shown me the secret nest, the rare bird, the wild thing scuttling across the track.' But they also enabled her to find sun while avoiding wind; to explore the footpaths, fields, streams and pubs that frequently flank lanes; and to reach 'the great high road which leads to the complicated city or . . . the cottage gate . . . or the church'. A meandering green lane takes you directly to civilisation. It is inherently sociable. You can amble or stride.

All of this appealed hugely to Tim Evans, a retired entrepreneur who began road walking in 2011 after reading about a 100 km cycling route through the Florida Keys. Tim has since clocked up over 20,000 km across much of Europe and the USA. 'I don't hike,' he told me. 'I road walk. I prefer paved routes. They go where I want to go, they are dry, flat and uniform, and pass through and by things I find interesting – the farms and cities and towns.' Tim walks roads and lanes because they make him feel connected to the world: 'I like civilisation,' he asserts. 'What I really like is to pick two places on a map and walk from one to the other. There's unlikely to be a hiking trail, but there'll always be a road.' Because Tim will pass places to eat, drink and sleep, he can travel with a mere two to three kilos of overnight kit, making his long walks less stressful: 'I feel as free as can be. Nowhere but on the open road is the body more unencumbered by belongings or the mind more free to roam without distractions.' For Tim, roads offer simplicity, convenience, conviviality, and a deep sense of purpose.

CHAPTER 3

"A meandering green lane takes you directly to civilisation"

'Few people walk with genuine purpose now,' he explains. 'They might go for a walk to get their steps up or to have a break from the city, for example, but we humans once walked to reach a useful destination. Road walking from town to town is how our ancestors moved. I feel as though I've tapped into a genetically coded drive – to keep moving, to keep discovering. I walk as other people drive – to get somewhere.'

Tim likes to think as he walks, and finds road walking highly conducive to contemplation, reflection and planning, invariably returning with his next route plotted out: 'When the walking and navigation is this easy, the mind can follow its own meandering paths.'

'People are often aghast when they hear that I prefer roads to wilderness trails,' he continues. 'But I've walked for days through the lanes of Britain, Spain and France – even parts of the United States – with barely any traffic at all.' Tim thinks that city dwellers make assumptions about the perils of traffic because they've never experienced the peace of a quiet leafy lane. 'City people assume that country roads are full of urban gridlocked traffic, but this isn't usually the case. Today, we think that roads are for vehicles and trails are for people and I find this very sad: it gives priority and precedence to machines, forcing humans into forests and mountains.' Tim points out that humans have walked from town to town along communal lanes for thousands of years. 'This landscape is our habitat – and it's being taken from us, yet another habitat destruction.'

Because roads have solid surfaces and are reliably free of impediments (bogs, bulls, broken bridges), Tim knows exactly how many kilometres he can walk each day (thirty, if you're asking), making the planning and timing of his walks easy and stress-free. With GPS and Google Maps downloaded onto his phone, he can find the quietest lanes, and the nearest pharmacy or shop. 'Walking lanes means I can sustain a good speed and rhythm, which is important when you're walking for transportation rather than recreation,' he adds.

Could walking with speed and rhythm be one of the reasons Tim finds such fulfilment in his lane walking? Quite possibly. Back in 2004, a Polish study pointed to the importance of rhythmic movement for alleviating anxiety and depression.[4] More recently, studies of older people have found rhythmic movement improves not only physical health (muscle strength, balance and flexibility) but quality of life.[5] According to Irish neuroscientist Shane O'Mara, the rhythm of walking induces 'all sorts of rhythms ... in the brain ... Rhythms that would previously be quiet suddenly come to life, and the way our brain interacts with our body changes.' He cites the rhythm of theta brainwaves – a frequency of 7–8 Hertz – which can be detected rolling over the brain as we walk, having amplified in order to help us navigate. O'Mara (a keen road walker) says one of the side effects of theta brainwaves is a greater ability to learn and remember.[6]

> "When the walking and navigation is this easy, the mind can follow its own meandering paths"

We know that walking more briskly reduces our chance of cancer, heart disease, dementia, osteoporosis and death,[7] but it may also improve our mood.[8] How so? When we move briskly our brain produces the hope molecule known as brain-derived neurotrophic factor (BDNF, see Introduction), a protein that promotes the growth of new neurons. Interestingly, BDNF appears to help recovery from depression and stress. In studies, depressed people often have lower concentrations of BDNF than their non-depressed counterparts. Movement raises our levels of BDNF.[9] And the brisker the movement, the more BDNF we produce.[10]

Recently, researchers have pinpointed a chain of biochemical interactions, known as the kynurenine pathway, for its critical role in mood disorders. Depressed people often have higher circulating levels of kynurenine, as do people with cancer, dementia, Parkinson's and heart disease. In fact, the more kynurenine in our blood, the greater our chances of dying sooner rather than later. Researchers speculate that inflammation activates an enzyme, causing our body to start making larger amounts of kynurenine, which in turn results in the formation and circulation of other damaging molecules in the body and brain.

Think of kynurenine as akin to household grease blocking up pipes. These blockages trigger a cascade effect of dangerous metabolites, shutting off much-needed pathways, including those that foster sleep (melatonin) and feelings of happiness (serotonin), much as a major blockage of grease in a kitchen pipe can cause downstream leaks in other parts of the house.

Unsurprisingly, pharmaceutical companies have been trying to make an anti-kynurenine drug for the last few years. They've not succeeded. But brisk, heart-pumping walking does exactly this, hindering the accumulation of kynurenine (and its toxic by-products) in our blood and tissues.

Could this explain why picking up the pace also appears to help us sleep better? In numerous studies, a faster pace has been linked with improved sleep. Slow-wave (deep) sleep appears to increase after 'moderate-intensity' movement,[11] as do levels of salivary melatonin.[12] In one experiment involving chronic insomniacs, a six-month programme of brisk movement 'yielded significant improvements in sleep health, quality of life, and mood', reported the authors, who also noted that the time of day made absolutely no difference.[13] So walk the lanes whenever you like.

Like kynurenine and BDNF, painkilling, feel-good endocannabinoids (which are now thought to cause the infamous runner's high) are also generated when we increase the intensity of our walk. What matters is effort (or intensity) rather than speed. Walking at a moderate speed but with great gusto is of more value than effortlessly running.[14]

While exerting effort makes us *feel* good, the accelerated speed enabled by a solid uniform surface also transforms our walk into a bone-building bonanza. For decades, running was deemed the only movement that could strengthen bones, along with weight and resistance training. Walking, said the bone experts, has little effect on preventing osteoporosis. In the last few years, new evidence has proven this wrong. Walking not only prevents bone loss but it can also fortify ageing bones, meaning fewer breakages and fractures. However, the walking must be fast and of a certain duration. When Dr Katarina Borer, an American professor of movement science, investigated the bone-mineral density of women pounding the tarmac pavements of a shopping mall, she found that a twenty-minute walk, however brisk, had little effect. 'What mattered was momentum (speed), and a duration of forty to forty-five minutes,' she told me, adding that the optimal walking speed was 6.3 km (four miles) per hour.

Tim has a name for his walking – free-route walking. 'Nothing beats seeing the world from the road, carrying only the bare essentials. You can't do that in the wilderness,' he says. But here's what I think about long-distance road walking: it's quite possibly the only way to unravel an entire *cultural landscape*. We walk the pretty lanes but we must also traverse the ugly roads. We cannot avoid the wastelands or suburbia. We uncover a place, warts and all, for better or worse – the overlooked orchids and hidden churches but also the forgotten apartment blocks and the decaying oil refineries. How else to fully understand the landscapes we humans have constructed?

notes

According to Tim Evans, the best places for lane walking are older, more densely populated areas where there are many rarely used roads that have been bypassed by newer highways. See www.roadwalking.com for maps and itineraries of Tim's walks in the US, Canada, Spain, France, Italy, Portugal, Switzerland, Belgium, Holland, Ireland and the UK.

Planning a long-distance road/lane walk? Forget the backpack. Tim wears a hiking waist (lumbar) pack containing only the bare essentials (also detailed on his website).

If there are no pavements or flat verges, you should walk facing oncoming traffic so that drivers can easily see you (with the exception of blind corners, when you might want to cross the road). Be prepared to walk single file, especially on narrow country roads or when the lighting is poor.

Your shoes should be comfortable and well padded, with a wide toe box and a lowish heel-to-toe drop. Carry a set of heel gels and blister plasters and consider wearing cushioned insoles inside your boot – the hard surface of lanes can take its toll if walking them day after day.

Take a walking pole (Tim uses a selfie stick) to wave at aggressive dogs who often 'guard' houses on country roads and are protective of their territory.

Moving to utter exhaustion raises levels of damaging kynurenine, so don't overdo it. A fast forty-five minutes is all you need for bone health, then slow it down to the three miles an hour recommended by walker and writer Rebecca Solnit as the ideal speed for thinking.

Unable to maintain your pace? Research shows that walking to a steady beat or music helps improve walking speed, stride length, walk rhythm and symmetry. Use a single earpiece to walk in time to some tunes, leaving the other ear for oncoming traffic.[15]

Note that some drivers use quiet country lines as a (misguided) chance to accelerate. Be prepared to tuck into the verge if need be.

If you're walking at dusk, wear a high-visibility tunic. Some road walkers advise wearing a high-vis band or layer at all times.

It's against the law (not to mention dangerous and unpleasant) to walk on major highways or motorways – keep to the leafy lanes and quiet country roads.

And finally, when calculating how far to walk, bear in mind that on hard, even surfaces, not only can we walk faster, we can also walk with greater mechanical efficiency (our muscles don't have to work as hard as when we're on sand, mud, scree, etc.), meaning we can often walk much further.

Rolling Hills

Resting the Eyes, Building the Body,
Settling the Mind

'[My] greatest pleasure in life was ... to roam on the heather-clad hills.'

FLORA THOMPSON, *HEATHERLEY*

— — — — — — — —

DEFINITION: A landscape of gently sloping hills, smaller than mountains but elevated above the surrounding land.

BENEFITS FOR: Fatigue, headaches, eye strain, myopia, glaucoma; an uneasy mind.

Over a century ago, an American psychologist called George Stratton sat and pondered the human predilection for curvature. He had a theory that our eyes are innately partial to curved lines because curved lines can be followed smoothly, continuously, effortlessly. Unlike sharp lines which – Stratton hypothesised – caused our eyes to move in uncomfortable and broken jerks, making it more difficult for our brain to process information along the way.

"Our eyes are innately partial to curved lines"

In 1975, long after Stratton had died, two researchers noted that four-week-old babies showed a preference for curved lines over sharp lines. They too speculated that the human visual system was, in some way, responsible for this instinctive preference. Thirty-five years later, another pair of researchers found that people detected the hidden details of curved polygons with greater speed than they spotted the hidden details of angular polygons. In other words, we humans process the information contained within curved lines more quickly and efficiently than that contained within sharp lines. Further experiments indicated that people were cognitively faster and more accurate when engaging with curved lines than when engaging with angled lines.[1]

Meanwhile, other studies found that curves were considered gentle and quiet while lines and angles were deemed agitating, hard and furious. Later experiments using neuroimaging technology revealed that curved and contoured objects and images caused less activity in the amygdala (our brain's threat-detection hub) than sharp objects and images. Experiments using fMRI found that participants preferred rounded rooms to angular rooms (particularly women, for whom the drop in subsequent stress was both marked and 'significant'[2]). Over and over again, smoothly rolling curves appear to make us happy.

"When we walk with exertion, our bodies produce a greater abundance of near-magical hope molecules"

Our eyes linger for longer on curves. We associate softly rounded shapes with comfort and pleasure (apparently).[3] They calm us. Indeed, neuroscientists have now identified the exact brain parts that respond preferentially to curvilinear contours. Little surprise, then, that in her bestselling memoir of burnout, Katherine May writes, 'Nothing settles my mind like a hill climb.'[4]

"Walking is most mood-lifting when it's brisk"

But our eyes' delight in the appealing undulations of hills isn't the only reason that an upward clamber can settle the mind. When we walk with exertion, our bodies produce a greater abundance of near-magical hope molecules.[5] Studies repeatedly tell us that movement is most restorative when it's moderately intense, that walking is most mood-lifting when it's brisk.

"A hill climb halts our ruminations"

Moreover, speeding up then slowing down (a version of high-intensity interval training, HIIT) is also particularly effective at prompting a flood of beautiful biochemicals while also giving us pause to recover. As a team of Mexican researchers put it, the most effective movement is that 'characterized by brief highly intense intervals'.[6] Which is exactly what happens when we puff our way up and down hills.

And yet there may be more at play than our walking-released biochemicals. Some researchers think the reason that a hill climb halts our ruminations is all down to the limited capacity of our working memory. When we feel anxious or depressed, our working memory becomes overloaded with the act of processing so much emotion. But when we walk with effort and puff, our working memory is subsumed by merely trying to get up the hill. 'Consequently there are fewer resources to devote to rumination,' stated a team of researchers after investigating the effects of short bursts of movement on rumination and mental health.[7] A hike of forty minutes was all it took – not enough time to climb a mountain, but perfectly adequate for a hill.

Having heaved our way, exultantly, to the top, other biological changes take place that bolster our wellbeing still further. At the summit, as we survey the panorama before us, our eyes switch into super-calming vista vision (see Chapter 18,

'Mountains'). But vista vision – where we look out as far as we can – is also excellent for our tired, screen-bound eyes. According to Andrew Huberman, neuroscientist and ophthalmologist, when we spend long hours 'focused on close-up objects – computers, screens, phones – the eye muscles and nerves that control them are working hard', exacerbating our near-sightedness (myopia). Huberman urges us to 'view far-off distances . . . throughout the day . . . beyond three feet out to infinity is key'.[8] Where better to gaze *out to infinity* than from a hilltop we have ascended on foot?

And yes, the ascent on foot matters. Why? Because intense movement seems to benefit our eyes as much as our body and brain. A recent study found that people doing moderately intense exercise had a lower risk of glaucoma,[9] while another report concluded that exercise has neuroprotective benefits on the retina. All of which is to say that a hill walk might be uniquely beneficial for our straining, twenty-first-century eyes.

"Space – it seems– can be genuinely transformative"

As we stand atop our hill, with our visual system in a splendid state of rest, we become startlingly aware of the space around us. This sense of space can also impact how we think and feel. A few years ago, psychologists investigating architectural space found intriguing associations between the space around us and our thoughts and emotions, even the moral decisions we make.

'Spaciousness influences emotion … and elicits more positive emotions,' they wrote in their report. This injection of positivity then alters the shape of our thoughts. The psychologists found that additional space made participants more tolerant and more empathetic. Small, tight spaces had the opposite effect, making participants feel more alone and more judgmental.[10] Being in a generously sized space makes us more open-minded and compassionate. Space – it seems – can be genuinely transformative.

This wasn't the first study to examine the effects of perceived space on our psyche. An earlier report had already suggested that high ceilings encouraged participants to think more conceptually and creatively, while low-slung ceilings helped participants to think in a way that was more empirical and detail-oriented.[11]

Philosopher Gaston Bachelard thought that people could be 'psychically innovated' in majestic spaces, and referred to 'vast' space as 'the friend of being', recognising that spaciousness brings with it sensations of freedom and opportunities for personal growth.[12] As we survey the world from the summit of our hill, warm and glowing from our ascent, the possibilities seem endless. Briefly, we are invincible.

"Walking up an incline forces our body to move against gravity"

Hill climbing is also a powerfully remedial form of movement for the body. When a team of American medics analysed stair-climbing data from over 450,000 people, whom they then followed for over twelve years, they found that the number of daily upwards steps was reflected in a reduced chance of getting coronary artery disease or having a stroke. In fact, people that climbed over fifty steps a day (the equivalent of hiking a few short inclines) cut their chances of heart disease by 20 per cent. Dr Lu Qi, one author of the study, told me that hill climbing would have exactly the same effect as stair-climbing, being 'vigorous exercise which can lower various risk factors for heart disease and can help in lowering body weight, improving metabolic health and inflammation'.[13]

How so? Walking either upstairs or up an incline forces our body to move against gravity. Our heart and lungs have to work harder. Indeed, hill climbing uses around three times as much energy as walking on the flat. But we also use different muscles, including those in our core and lower back – making a hill walk particularly good for our waistline, our sense of balance and our lower spine.

Nor is it all about going uphill. The downhill is equally valuable: we use different muscles when we descend – making hill walking an excellent means of reaching every chain of lower-body muscles. More recently, downhill walking has been identified as particularly beneficial for building stronger bones, helping fend off frailty and osteoporosis. When Dr Katarina Borer examined the role of walking in bone health, she found that both fast and downhill walking had a marked effect on bone-mineral density.[14]

Unlike mountains, hills are everywhere. Their height and gradient are less intimidating than mountains. We don't need special kit. We don't need a head for heights. Hills really are for everyone. And yet – exactly like a mountain – hills have a summit that quietly urges us upwards and onwards. Here, our mind, body and the landscape itself momentarily connect, all of us in an upwards trajectory of hope and purpose.

notes

Look out for cols – gaps or depressions in a ridge or between hills, often formed from glaciation or tectonic movement. According to Graham Robb, cols were once renowned for their 'magical qualities'.[15]

Always zig-zag your way up a hill. The straight, direct path is only the most energetically efficient if the gradient of the hill is less than 14° (a gentle incline). Studies indicate that we humans tend to go for the most direct route, despite it being the least biologically efficient. But for any gradient above 14°, we minimise our energy expenditure by zig-zagging.[16]

Hills are not just for the countryside: seek out hilly cities like Lisbon, Edinburgh and San Francisco. Avoid public transport and enjoy heart-thumping views that will soothe your frazzled nerves, tone your leg and abdominal muscles, improve your eye health and strengthen your heart.

From your hilltop, feast your eyes on meandering rivers and curving paths. According to Dr Marc Berman, director of Chicago University's Environmental Neuroscience Lab, curvy landscape features relax us: 'We evolved with them,' he explains, and so they are 'processed more fluently by the brain'.[17]

ROLLING HILLS

Hills are often the sites of prehistoric remains, from Bronze Age forts to standing stones. Go to Chapter 12, 'Therapeutic Landscapes' for more on ancient and magical landscapes.

The benefits of hill walking aren't restricted to heart, lung and brain health: according to Dr James Hotaling, an expert in urology, 'walking up a steep hill [is one] of the few things that will increase endogenous testosterone production'.[18]

Want something more ambitious? Chapter 18 covers the curative powers of mountains.

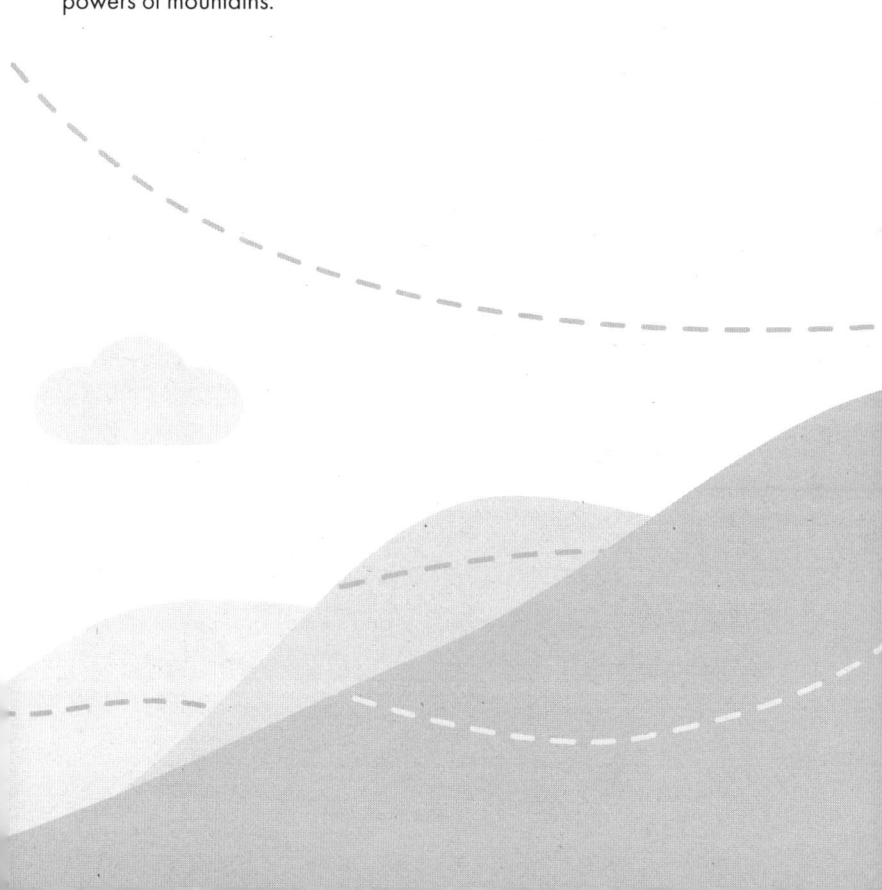

Cemeteries

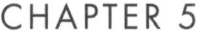

Lessons in Mortality

'During the lockdown, the cemetery behind my house became a sanctuary. I walked there most days . . . I found it a vaccine against gloom.'

PETER ROSS, *A TOMB WITH A VIEW*

DEFINITION: An area set apart for graves and tombs. From the Greek, 'sleeping chamber'.

BENEFITS FOR: Fear of mortality and death, sadness, those in need of sanctuary or a renewed sense of gratitude, loneliness.

When author Clare Pooley was diagnosed with breast cancer, her first thought was for her children. 'They were six, eight and eleven, and I wanted them to know, but I didn't want them to worry,' she said as we ambled through London's Brompton Cemetery. 'So I told them that everything was going to be all right.' Clare's decision meant that she had to maintain a demeanour of calm and confidence at home. 'And yet I was frightened and sad. Crying was very therapeutic for me, but I couldn't cry at home in case my children saw me.' Clare isn't religious, but she began walking and crying in her local cemetery, explaining that 'a cemetery is the one place where we expect to see people crying. Walking between gravestones gave me permission to express emotions I couldn't express anywhere else. These moments of teary but much-needed decompression became a sort of emotional detox.'

As Clare walked round her local cemetery, she began reading the gravestones. 'It became a place of stories – some were sad, others were intriguing, and many were inspiring. I read the names, ages and epitaphs, even the Bible quotes, and wondered about the hundreds of lives that had gone before me,' she explained. 'This made me feel incredibly grateful for my own life, for the fact that none of my children had died as babies. I knew that most of the women – often footnotes on their husbands' graves – had experienced much harder and shorter lives than mine. Suddenly I was overwhelmed with gratitude.'

Walking in a cemetery every day gave Clare a sense of perspective. 'The old headstones were a visual representation of all the lives that had gone before mine, and this gave me a powerful sense of temporal perspective. My life was just one in a long chain. And because the cemetery was so peaceful and felt quite spiritual, I could reflect on this in a way I couldn't anywhere else.'

As Clare slowly recovered, the significance of the cemetery changed. 'I started noticing different things – the birds and trees, for example. But I also began seeking out the inspiring graves – the people who had achieved something. I now knew that life was potentially short and if I wanted to achieve something, I had to get on with it.' The cemetery became a source of inspiration, just as it had for Beatrix Potter who, 150 years earlier, had found names for some of her best-known characters on headstones. 'I started work on my first novel, *The Authenticity Project*, and the cemetery became one of the book's most important locations,' Clare tells me. Today, many of Clare's readers make pilgrimages to Brompton Cemetery.

I share Clare's passion for walking in cemeteries. Here we must confront our own mortality. And while mountains and plains give us a vital sense of spatial perspective, nowhere gifts us a greater sense of temporal perspective than a cemetery. Among the headstones of history, we see ourselves as we are – a fleeting moment in the endless passage of time, a cluster of cells that, like everything else, will one day return to the earth. Whether we return from a cemetery walk with a feeling of gratitude, awash in gentle melancholy, or with a fresh sense of purpose, is up to us.

Psychologists now recognise that the signalling of a space also plays a role. Which is to say that having places designed for, or specifically acknowledging, grief might be more important than previously thought. 'Walking in a place associated with sadness tells our brain that loss is normal, that we have taken our first steps of recovery – and this seems to be as important as the space itself,' grief therapist Sarah O'Hara told me.

Whenever I travel, I walk the local cemeteries and churchyards. In fact, they are often the first places I visit, because they act as windows into the culture and history of communities. The travel writer and actress Nancy Price did exactly the same thing back in the 1950s, writing, 'My first visit is to the church wherever my wanderings take me. I find it the best guide to the history of the place.'[1] In Brussels, in 1853, when the writer Charlotte Brontë was at her loneliest, she would walk the local cemetery (she called it 'a pilgrimage') to assuage her feelings of isolation.[2]

"An aura of spirituality adds to the contemplative and healing nature of these places"

Neither I, Clare Pooley, Charlotte Brontë nor Nancy Price are unusual in this. Nor are we the first to recognise the balm-like effect of 'cities of the dead' on our minds. Indeed, we are part of a large community sometimes called taphophiles, or tombstone tourists.

"Cemeteries blend past and future, life and death, material and spiritual, heaven and Earth"

Recently, a handful of researchers started studying the restorative effects of spiritual spaces. Churches, monasteries and convents have been found to offer many of the mind-quietening benefits more usually associated with nature.[3] A few environmental psychologists have started drawing our attention to the importance of spaces deemed 'spiritual', finding that an aura of spirituality adds to the contemplative and healing nature of these places, regardless of whether they are 'green', 'blue' or plain brown.*

"The cities of the dead are windows into every aspect of humanity"

Cemetries go a step further – not only can we walk them, but they brilliantly blend past and future, life and death, material and spiritual, heaven and Earth, the natural with the architectural, the cultural with the sacred. When we walk a cemetery, we are plunged into an enthralling blend of greenery and history, wild space and cultural space. Here, rare plants sit alongside quirks of art and architecture. Man-made icons of time rub shoulders with

---

* Green, blue and brown space are the terms typically used by researchers to denote planted/leafy (green) spaces, water-dominated (blue) spaces, or urban/built (brown) spaces.

songbirds and butterflies. Mourners, dog walkers, pilgrims and the merely curious cross paths – all of them companioned by the rich vein of stories carved into hundreds (sometimes thousands) of headstones. As Yolanda Zappaterra wrote in her book *Cities of the Dead: The World's Most Beautiful Cemeteries*, 'The cities of the dead are windows into every aspect of humanity and its nature. Here, laid bare, are clearly visible mankind's potential for greatness – intelligence, personal achievements, philanthropy, generosity, creativity, imagination – but also our potential for weakness and failure – bloodlust, war, famine, greed and brutality.'[4]

Cemeteries do more than distract us with their stories. They remind us that the human experience of loss, recovery and remembrance is universal; it is the single experience that connects us all. This is a therapeutic landscape like no other.

"Cemeteries foster relaxation, reflection and contemplation"

For decades, cemeteries lay outside the remit of academic study. Many were seen merely as real estate, destined for developers. Others were considered creepy or reminders of a past no one wanted to confront. But in the last few years cemeteries have become the subject of numerous psychological studies from as far afield as Norway, Hungary, Scotland, Finland, Denmark, Turkey, Kuala Lumpur and North America. Cemetery walkers have been interviewed in detail, their emotions recorded, analysed and compared. Most researchers agree – these are peaceful places providing emotional restitution. 'Cemeteries foster relaxation, reflection and contemplation,' wrote Professor Helena Nordh, after interviewing cemetery walkers in Oslo.[5]

"This is a therapeutic landscape like no other"

Government, councils and researchers are finally taking note of the extraordinary opportunities offered by cemeteries. In 2010 the Council of Europe announced a new Cemeteries Route – a map identifying over sixty historically and ecologically important cemeteries spread over twenty countries. More are being added all the time. 'These sacred and emotional spaces,' stated the Council, 'are witnesses of local history for cities and towns.' 'Our cemeteries,' they explained, reveal the cultural and religious identity of a place, adding: 'It is important to see cemeteries as places of life.'[6]

More recently, cemeteries have been lauded as vital green spaces, havens of urban wildlife in the heart of ever-denser cities. When researchers monitored the wildlife of Berlin's Jewish Weißensee cemetery, they were stunned to find more than 604 species, of which ten were either rare or protected.[7] Bats, birds, lichens, mosses, beetles, spiders, plants and trees had been largely undisturbed for decades. Meanwhile, ecologists tallying plant life in sacred sites situated across one of India's largest metropolises logged over 121 species, concluding that these places 'play an important role in urban biodiversity conservation'.

It isn't only urban cemeteries that are preserving biodiversity. When rural cemeteries were surveyed, they too were harbouring wildlife that had largely been eliminated from surrounding farmland. Cemeteries in Australia and the United States were found to have rare grassland species, Turkish and German cemeteries were home to orchids, while Polish cemeteries contained woodland plants no longer found in the adjacent fields.[8] Rural cemeteries, it appears, provide habitat islands for native species that have been eradicated from intensively farmed rural landscapes.

Cemeteries should be walked slowly. Indeed, if we're to reflect or to read and ponder the stories inscribed on headstones, we cannot go at a brisk pace. No matter. New research suggests that a slow, contemplative pace is more physiologically beneficial than previously thought. When Andrew Agbaje, a researcher at the University of Eastern Finland, studied 800 young adults, he found that the amount of vigorous activity they did hadn't changed over time. But their 'light physical activity' had declined by 3.5 hours a day. During this – increasingly sedentary – time, their levels of inflammation had doubled (in fact it had tripled in young women). Agbaje was surprised to see that the more body fat participants had, the less effective was vigorous exercise at reducing inflammation. But this wasn't the case for light physical activity – strolling and pottering, for instance. 'Light physical activity appears to be the key to almost universal success regarding health,' Agbaje commented, adding that this sort of gentle movement might just be 'an unsung hero'.[9]

Clare Pooley agrees that cemeteries are the perfect place to potter: 'All those headstones of people who died at a much younger age than mine reminded me that every new day I have is a day to celebrate. I wouldn't have seen them if I'd been striding or marching . . .'

In a cemetery, we amble, pause, bend, stoop, kneel. Nor does it matter how long we walk for. When we're sad or depressed, even twenty minutes can make a difference. When Dr Eamon Laird, a research fellow at Trinity College Dublin, studied the activities and states of mind of 4,000 adults aged fifty and over, he was astonished at the effects of a twenty-minute walk. 'As little as twenty minutes of daily walking, five days a week, appeared to cut the risk of depression by up to 43 per cent,' he explained. And if they walked for longer, even better. Laird's ten-year study showed that the risk of depression fell in proportion to the time spent walking. 'But for many people, twenty minutes was all it took to make a difference to their mood. We hadn't expected such a dramatic result,' he added.[10]

notes

There are many wonderful books on exploring cemeteries. For the world traveller, Yolanda Zappaterra's *Cities of the Dead* contains information on some of the most memorable burial sites on the planet. For the UK, I like Peter Ross's *A Tomb With a View: The Stories and Glories of Graveyards* and Ann Treneman's *Finding the Plot: 100 Graves to Visit Before You Die*.

Look out for cemeteries offering guided tours and even night 'ghost walks'.

CHAPTER 5

Wherever you are, chances are there's a burial site on your doorstep – a church graveyard, cemetery, standing stones, or something else altogether.

War-memorial parks and remembrance gardens provide similarly reflective places in which to walk and contemplate.

Cemeteries often attract solo walkers, and most are places of peace and quiet, often with dog-free and cycle-free paths, making them ideal for walkers in search of urban solitude.

Some of my favourite cemeteries include Prague's Jewish cemeteries, London's famous Magnificent Seven Victorian cemeteries, Paris's Père Lachaise and Montmartre cemeteries, Rome's Protestant Graveyard and Turin's Cimitero Monumentale. Zappaterra's favourites include the cemeteries of New Orleans, Kolkata's South Park Cemetery (India), Venice's Isola di San Michele, Mount Auburn in Cambridge, Massachusetts, Green-Wood in Brooklyn, New York, and the coastal Waverley in Sydney, Australia.

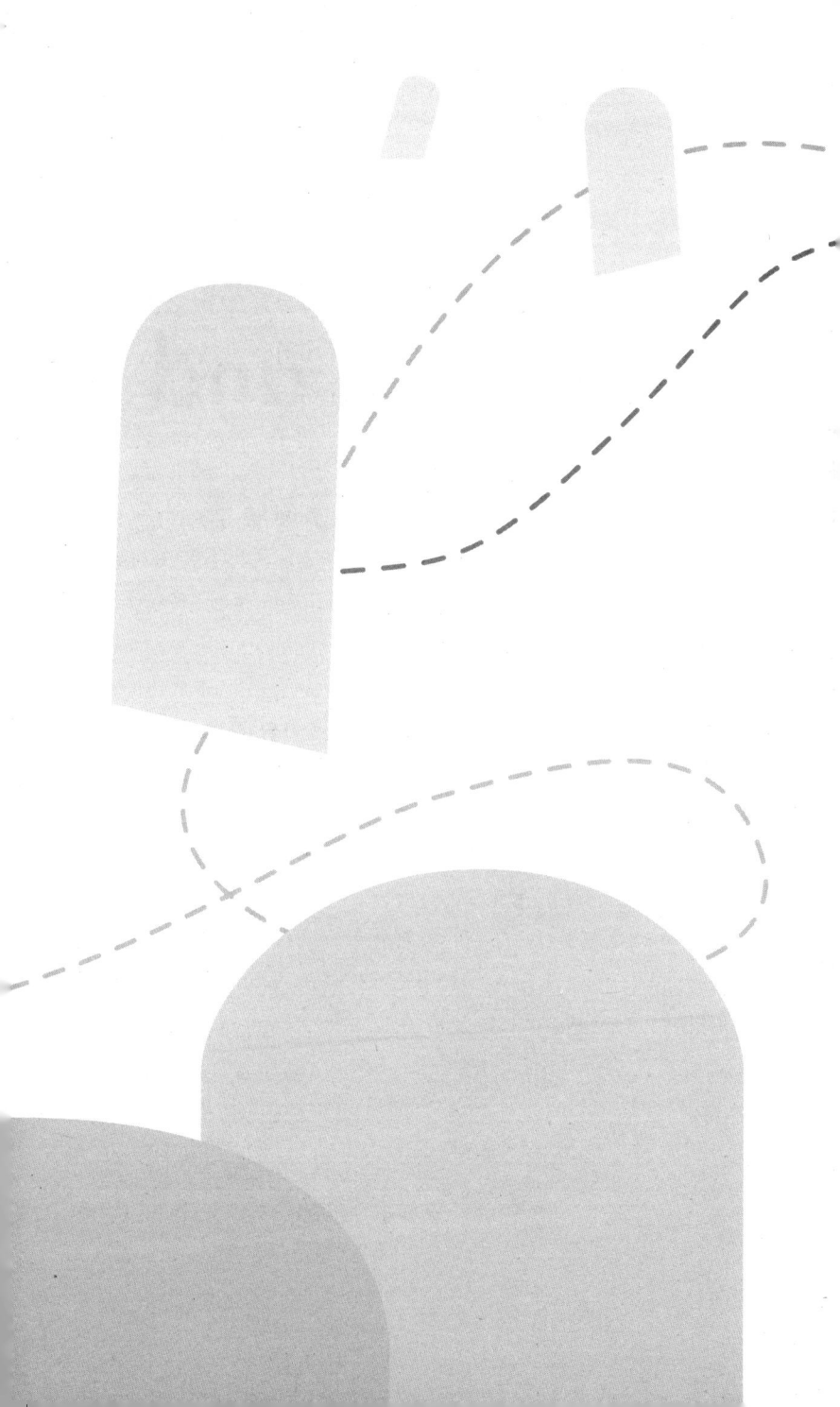

Flowers and Meadows

The Astonishing Alchemy of
Aromatic Landscapes

'It seemed to me, when I have been walking [in these Alpine valleys], as if every flower I ever saw in a garden met me somewhere in the rocks or meadows . . . A continued exhalation of joy.'

HARRIET BEECHER STOWE, *SUNNY MEMORIES OF FOREIGN LANDS*

DEFINITION: Flower-rich grassland of all types.

BENEFITS FOR: Forgetfulness, fear of memory loss, anxiety.

CHAPTER 6

'I am like a dog – smell excites me,' wrote walker and writer Nan Shepherd in her celebrated paean to the Scottish mountains, *The Living Mountain*. 'All the aromatic and heady fragrances – pine and birch, bog myrtle, the spicy juniper, heather and the honey-sweet orchis, and the clean smell of wild thyme . . . are there to be smelled,' she says before urging us to go out and sniff, to grub up the earth, to plunge our nose into grass, moss and wild berry bushes.

Shepherd knew instinctively what scientists are finally proving – that smell can exert a powerful influence on our mind and our mood, on how we feel, think and remember. Researchers now think that essential-oil molecules, once inhaled, travel directly to the brain, where they help create new brain cells, regulate our hormones, and favourably alter the chemistry of our blood. They also activate certain brain regions, particularly our memory powerhouse, the hippocampus, and our fear-and-emotion hub, the amygdala. The chemicals with these magic effects on mood and memory – linalool, limonene, benzyl benzoate, benzyl alcohol, β-pinene – are currently being isolated and studied in laboratories, with astounding results.[1]

"Smell can exert a powerful influence on our mind and our mood"

Lavender and chamomile have proven to ease symptoms of depression, anxiety and stress in adults of all ages. In tests, lavender lowers blood pressure and reduces anxiety. Some oils – ylang ylang, bergamot, lemon – appear to raise levels of feel-good serotonin and dopamine. Cinnamon oil seems to inhibit pro-inflammatory cytokines. Orange, rose and lavender reduce levels of the stress-related hormone, cortisol, circulating in our blood. Musk, lemon and rosemary are associated with a greater production of brain-derived neurotrophic factor (BDNF), a protein that helps maintain healthy brain cells.[2] Plants – and particularly perfumed flowers – can biochemically alter us, making us calmer and happier.

But that's not all. Neurobiologist Dr Michael Leon recently published a study in which participants exposed to a rota of seven different essential oils (peppermint, rose, eucalyptus, rosemary, orange, lemon and lavender) for two hours a day achieved a jaw-dropping 226 per cent improvement in memory, when compared to a control group.[3] Functional magnetic resonance imaging (fMRI) revealed that participants exposed to the odours had strengthened and expanded a brain region linked to memory and cognition, known as the uncinate fasciculus.

'The olfactory system is the only sense that has a direct "superhighway" input to the memory centers of the brain; all the other senses have to reach those brain areas through what you might call the brain's "side streets", and so they have much less impact on maintaining the health of those memory centers,' Dr Leon told Medscape Medical News. When our sense of smell weakens, 'The memory centers of the brain start to deteriorate and, conversely, when people are [exposed to diverse odours], their memory areas become larger and more functional,' he explained. Leon calls this 'olfactory enrichment' and believes it's vital to healthy ageing, adding that loss of smell is often a first symptom of Alzheimer's disease.

"Our olfactory cells resemble muscles – use them or lose them"

But loss of smell also accompanies most neurological and psychiatric disorders. 'I've counted sixty-eight of them – including anorexia, anxiety, ADHD, depression, epilepsy and stroke,' Leon said,[4] adding that, by midlife, our risk of dying can be predicted by our ability to smell. Leon speculates that the modern world may have left us chronically bereft of the high levels of olfactory stimulation we evolved with, and that a brain deprived of olfactory stimulation and with a weakened ability to smell is somehow more vulnerable to the symptoms of mental and neurological illness.[5]

And yet we don't need to lose our sense of smell. Our olfactory cells resemble a muscle – use them or lose them. And the more we use them, the better our brains. In 2022, researchers recruited a group of sommelier students, who are typically exposed to dozens of new smells every day as part of their training. The students had their brains scanned at the beginning and end of their eighteen-month training programme, and the scans were then compared to those of a control group. To the researchers' surprise, not only did the sommelier students have a much larger olfactory bulb, but their eighteen months of training resulted in a much thicker entorhinal cortex, which meant improved memory and recall. The control group, however, experienced no changes in either their ability to detect smell or their brain.[6]

We don't have to be healthy young sommeliers to grow our smell muscle. In a study published at the same time, older adults with moderate dementia who were exposed to forty scents twice a day for just over two weeks showed significant improvements in memory, mood, ability to concentrate and verbal dexterity.[7]

Take a moment to imagine this profusion of mind-altering perfumes mixing, merging and melding with the cocktail of hope molecules precipitated when we walk (see Introduction). It's a mind-boggling thought – the magical medicine of movement compounded and amplified by the extraordinary sorcery of plant oils.

But where can we find such scent-rich, aromatic landscapes? Plants release aromatic volatile compounds (1,700 have been identified to date) in order to attract pollinators, deter herbivores, 'talk' to other plants, and as protection against excessive light, temperature and oxidative stress. In other words, an aromatic landscape is dense with perfumed plant life. Using essential oils may be an easy shortcut, but nothing beats an amble through the full panoply of odours we find in scented spaces. As olfactory researchers have noted, an oil is only as good as the chemicals preserved within it. In their natural habitat, these chemicals reach us purely, directly and at no cost.

Even a simply planted garden of grass, lavender, pansies and a few willows has been found to have high levels of several phytoncides including phenol (an antioxidant and anti-inflammatory compound), benzaldehyde (anti-cancerous) and benzoic acid (antimicrobial).[8]

Most studies of botanical fragrances have been done in laboratories using essential oils. But in the Swedish rehabilitation garden, Alnarp, researchers decided to explore the effects of a living smellscape on mental health. Working with fifty-nine patients suffering from stress, exhaustion, burnout, anxiety and depression, the Alnarp team spent five years studying the effects of plant perfumes on mood.

"Odour had more impact on stress reduction than either visual or auditory stimuli"

Patients commented regularly on the comfort of fragrance: rosemary, lavender, verbena, straw, the smell of earth, hay, grass. One odour was deemed to be particularly consoling and uplifting – geranium (pelargonium), with a variety known as Dr Westerlund being repeatedly highlighted.[9] Not only did patients report a greater, scent-amplified connection to nature, but they noted that using their sense of smell had made them feel more embodied, helping them disconnect from their intellect. The Alnarp researchers remarked that odour had more impact on stress reduction than either visual or auditory stimuli.

It's not only smell that determines our mood while walking in an aromatic landscape. Patients in the Alnarp garden also pointed out that colour schemes were important. They appreciated well-balanced planting schemes 'consisting of soft colours in the flowerbeds, and soft structure of plants . . . no odd or bright colours or hard shapes'. In the early part of their treatment, when participants were at their most emotionally exhausted, bright colours and severe or angular designs were too tiring.

As the rehabilitation programme progressed, participants felt better equipped to appreciate bright flowers. Then – but only then – could the brilliance of the blooms bring cheer and joy. 'In the beginning of the rehabilitation period the participants were in need of a soft colour scheme,' explained Dr Pálsdóttir. 'But later, as their mental and physical power increased, they could handle stronger colours . . . red or bright yellow and orange.'

Studies of flower colour have found heart rates were noticeably affected by hue, increasing in the presence of red and yellow blooms. In addition, the results suggested that, regardless of the degree of whiteness, the hue had a significant impact on participants' emotions; blue increased relaxation and calmness compared to other colours.[10]

When researchers at Tongji University's College of Architecture and Urban Planning ran an experiment comparing the mood of employees in an office with flowers to those in a flower-less office, the results were clear. Those with daily access to flowers reported greater feelings of calm, cheerfulness and solace, more marked when the flowers were blue. The researchers concluded that flowering plants were 'a promising therapeutic approach for enhancing physiological functions and improving psychological relaxation for office workers'.[11]

"In the presence of flowers, people stood more closely to one another"

But do the flower effects last or are they merely a flash in the pan? Professor Jeannette Haviland-Jones decided to investigate with a series of experiments. The results took her by surprise: Even a single flower appeared to change human behaviour for the better. 'It is possible that flowers – either through their visual or odorous qualities – have [enduring] effects on brain chemistry,' she noted.

Among her more unexpected findings was that flowers 'closed the distance between strangers'.[12] In the presence of flowers, people stood more closely to one another, spoke and smiled more readily.

How to explain this? Haviland-Jones wondered if humans had acquired a 'learned association of flowers with positive social events'. But equally, she noted, we may connect flowers with survival, courtesy of an evolutionary response in which flowers indicated the presence of nuts, seeds, edible roots and leaves. Flowers, she speculated, have evolved as 'human sensory mood enhancers'. In which case, we're biologically primed to enjoy flowers, because our distant ancestors associated their beauty with the welcome relief of finding food. Which is to say, the colours, textures, shapes and perfumes of flowers calm us.

Haviland-Jones also noticed that we move differently in the presence of flowers. Whether wild or in a vase, flowers render us embodied. We stoop or stretch to sniff and examine them. We move foliage to find them. We touch them, pick them, arrange them. We sigh over their exquisite symmetries. Flowers make us feel safe, companioned, grateful for their undemanding beauty.

notes

Flowers pollinated by bees and butterflies usually release their scents in the day, while those pollinated by moths and bats do so from dusk onwards. Take an evening walk to catch these sweet perfumes at their headiest.

Walk in your scented landscape as often as you can: researchers found that daily thirty-minute exposure to scents, when done for three months, induced neurogenesis in the olfactory bulb and the hippocampus (both the ability to smell and to recall improved).

Evergreen forests are highly aromatic (see Chapter 1), particularly on warm days. Meanwhile, many of the most popular garden flowers are also high in terpenes and terpenoids, including jasmine, chrysanthemum, roses and lilies, all of which have – in studies – evoked feelings of serenity and joy.[13]

Don't pick (or step on) flowers, but do smell them and do rub/bruise the leaves of herbs (and geraniums) to release their aroma. Scents linger in dips and valleys, so look for sheltered scent-scapes.

Touching petals, leaves and bark also enriches our skin microbiota, improving our immunity. In a study of children, those handling soil and greenery every day showed enhanced skin microbiota and greater resistance to illness.[14]

Seek out herb gardens, lavender, rose and tulip farms that are open to the public. Visit scented gardens like those at the Cambridge University Botanic Garden, the International Perfume Museum in Grasse, France and the Perfumer's Garden in Versailles, near Paris. Bluebell woods combine tree and flower phytoncides, while pick-your-own farms often have blackcurrant bushes, the leaves and buds of which contain abundant, health-enhancing terpenes. Just scratch 'n' sniff!

Researchers have found that when smells noted while walking are re-experienced later on, people can more clearly recall the original occasion than those who walked without actively smelling. To remember your walk, choose a scented location, and close your eyes and ears intermittently to get the full perfume effect.

No flowers nearby? The smell of green (leaves, grass) might be as powerful. A 2009 experiment involving stressed rodents found that scents conjured from leaves had a remarkably calming effect, reducing bloods levels of a wide range of stress-related compounds.[15]

City Strolling

The Energising Excitement of a Walkable City

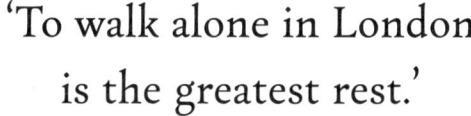

'To walk alone in London
is the greatest rest.'

VIRGINIA WOOLF, *STREET HAUNTING*

DEFINITION: A relatively permanent and highly
organised centre of population, of greater size or
importance than a town or village.

BENEFITS FOR: Boredom, lethargy, restlessness,
cravings for both solitude and human connection,
'bad feelings'.

Lately it has become fashionable to lambast our cities as places to walk: too noisy, too crowded, too polluted, too dangerous. And while I agree that walking in a thick cloud of air pollution, or pushing our way along crowded pavements accompanied by a thrum of traffic, is rarely conducive to lung health, serenity or calm, I happen to love urban walking. I love the unexpected encounters with strangers. I love the endless variations: a city at dawn is nothing like a city at night; a city in rain or snow is nothing like a city on a hot summer's day. And I love the opportunities for surprise – the backstreets and byways, the forgotten bars and bistros, the tucked-away markets and hidden architecture, the weeds that bloom from cracks and crevices. They may not always soothe our frazzled, fractured nerves, but all good cities should stimulate and entertain us.

"It is in cities that our collective creativity and ingenuity is most manifest"

Which is why, whenever I'm feeling bored or restless, whenever I need jolting out of lethargy, I head to the city. Whenever I want to be so distracted that I no longer care *who* or *how* I am, I head to the city. Whenever I want to walk alone without feeling alone, I head to the city. Whenever I want to feel deeply connected to my own species, I head to the city. Here I can wander among the very best of my fellow humans' achievements – for it is in cities that our collective creativity and ingenuity is most manifest. From churches to art galleries, from bakeries to urban graffiti, every city carries a fingerprint of aspiration and imagination.

> "Environments in which we feel safe and comfortable place fewer processing demands on our brains"

I'm not unusual: when Professor Opitz used brain-scanning technology to measure responses to cities versus countryside, he found that both landscapes elicited feelings of happiness in equal measure, but while green space was more likely to calm us, cities made us feel excited.

For all their exuberance, urban spaces can also feel

reassuringly familiar, thanks to their easily navigable streets and the plentiful presence of other people. In fact, when it comes to walking, what often matters most is *how safe* we feel. When researchers from Bristol University analysed the gait of walkers in both urban and rural locations, they found that both groups shifted their gait – walking more cautiously and less steadily – as they became less comfortable. This shift of gait happened as much on nature walks as on urban walks. 'Environments in which we feel safe and comfortable place fewer processing demands on our brains,' explains psychologist Daria Burtan.[1]

When we have fewer demands on our brains, we are granted the cognitive time and space to attend to the details around us and to fully revel in our walk. In the city that includes bending our ear to its many sounds and smelling its many odours, as well as people-watching, museum-hopping and window-shopping.

So perhaps it's no surprise that solo female walkers often prefer sauntering in busy cities to hiking through less peopled rural areas. Indeed, dozens of women have written effusively of their urban ambles, finding in them a sense of anonymity, creativity and liberation.

'In Paris,' wrote Russian artist Marie Bashkirtseff in her diary, 'everything interests me; instead of being lazy, I am in too great a hurry. I should like not only to walk, but to fly.' Greta Garbo loved walking the streets of New York – which she did twice daily for forty years. When asked what her future plans were, having not made a film for years, she replied, 'I walk. That's what I'm doing. I walk.' Garbo liked to stroll in and out of antique stores, to peer through shop windows, to visit markets and browse art galleries. In her oversized dark glasses, she walked the same streets – from the east end of 52nd Street, where she lived, up and down First, Second and Third Avenues – never tiring of the sights, smells and sounds of New York City.

For New Zealand writer Janet Frame, walking the streets of London ('by myself . . . looking at buildings') was an endless source of creative material. 'It probably looks like I'm doing nothing,' she said of her daily stroll. 'However, on these walks, things just come into my mind.'

No one expresses the therapeutic joys of city strolls better than American author Vivian Gornick. In her essay 'On the Street', Gornick describes how a daily walk effectively purges her of 'bad feeling', writing, 'Nothing heals me of a sore and angry heart like a walk through the city . . . never am I less alone than alone in the crowded street.' By 'walking slowly' among 'the endlessly advancing crowd', Gornick feels herself revived and energised: 'Within a mile my pace quickens, my eyes relax, my ears clear out . . . my shoulders straighten, my stride lengthens. The misery in my chest begins to dissolve . . . I feel free.'

Here we have it: in cities, our 'bad feeling', 'misery' and fatigue are swiftly elbowed out, *purged*, by unending colour and diversion. This bountiful distraction is why many environmental psychologists believe urban walking is less emotionally restorative than rural walking. On city walks, our brains must work overtime to keep us safe from traffic and other pedestrians, to resist the lure of constant consumption, to record the novel and unfamiliar. How on earth can we be expected to decompress in a city?

"Cities can calm, comfort, distract and inspire us"

And yet, in the last few years, a small group of researchers have begun questioning the idea that only nature can restore our jaded spirits. If we humans have lived for centuries in communities and amid buildings and markets, they ask, why are urban parks the only city space deemed restorative? In 2017 a team of Spanish researchers decided to investigate the effects of walking in 'the built environment'. They were particularly curious about the influence of squares (piazzas, plazas), and identified two for their experiment – one full of greenery and one containing scant greenery but with bars, shops and a church. Forty-six tired, stressed participants were then surveyed before, during and after walking for thirty minutes round the two squares. Both groups demonstrated improved concentration, greater happiness and reduced tension, anxiety, anger and fatigue. But – to the researchers' surprise – those in the more built-up square reported higher energy levels and a much greater reduction in stress than those in the abundantly green square.[2]

Since then, several other studies have found that walking through a city's historic quarters prompts profound feelings of calm.[3] In fact, recent research using fMRI suggests that temples, churches, courtyards and beautiful contemporary buildings are particularly adept at rewiring our brains, making us feel 'connected, transported, appreciative, intensely absorbed, and yet calm and relaxed ... a meditative state induced by contemplative architecture'.[4] Like lushly green spaces, historic cities and the very best of modern design can calm, comfort, distract and inspire us.[5]

We may even walk differently in cities. While in Venice, the sculptor Barbara Hepworth was struck by the way walkers responded to the proportions of the city's architectural spaces: 'They walked differently, discovering their innate dignity. They grouped themselves in unconscious recognition of their importance in relation to each other as human beings.'[6] A beautiful city, she reminds us, can do as much for our *innate dignity* as any other deeply satisfying landscape.

notes

Seek out walkable cities – for me this means non-sprawling cities with ample pavements, plenty of pedestrianised areas and minimal air pollution. No one wants to breathe diesel as they stroll.

Studies[7] suggest that the two things we like least about city walking are the noise and the pollution – use an air-quality index app to check pollution levels before your walk. I use AirVisual, which monitors levels of both particulate matter and other pollutants, such as nitrogen dioxide, in most of the world's cities.

After cross-referencing dozens of studies, I've found the world's most enjoyably walkable cities to be (at the time of writing): Zurich, Stockholm, Sydney, Vancouver and Tallinn. Closer to home, Edinburgh, Glasgow and Liverpool consistently have low rates of air pollution (alongside lots to see), while St Albans has more walking routes than any other UK city.

While the top most walkable cities tend to be in Europe, a 2024 survey reported in *Forbes* included Boston, Istanbul, Melbourne, Jersey City, Shanghai and Toronto.[8]

Look for historic cities: old buildings, open pedestrianised spaces and cultural landmarks please us most – but bear in mind these are often the busiest cities. Walk out of season or early in the morning to beat the crowds and traffic.

Use a green-walking app like GoJauntly to avoid stress-inducing arterial roads – where our cognitive capacities are consumed by having to stay safe. Incidentally, a growing body of research links traffic pollution with a greater risk of depression. Neuroimaging studies have also found that an overdose of pollution changes the structure of certain brain parts among children and adolescents.[9] If you live in a city, lobby for traffic restrictions.

On hot days, avoid narrow, high-rise streets, where a lack of circulation can make the air both stale, polluted and overly hot.[10] When temperatures climb, look for shady, tree-lined streets and squares.

Look for less crowded areas: studies consistently show that navigating busy places requires far more vigilance, overloading our minds still further.

Cities are at their least polluted after rainfall and at quiet times like dawn. Walk as far from the edge of the road as you can, avoid rush hour and gridlocked, slow-moving traffic.

Slow down: a faster pace with its increased respiration also means more harmful particulate matter (and other pollutants) entering our lungs.

Seek out the unseen and the unnoticed, the parts and places that don't make it into guidebooks or TripAdvisor reviews. Turn to Chapter 16, 'Outlands' to find out why the unexpected will always thrill us more than the things we've seen in guidebooks or on social media.

Want to combine city sights with a good workout? Opt for hilly cities like Porto, San Francisco and Edinburgh.

Craving greenery? Most historic cities have a river (see Chapter 19), canal (see Chapter 13), cemeteries (see Chapter 5), parks and gardens (see Chapter 15).

Irritated that your own city feels unwalkable? Join (or start) a local group campaigning to make your city more pedestrian-friendly.

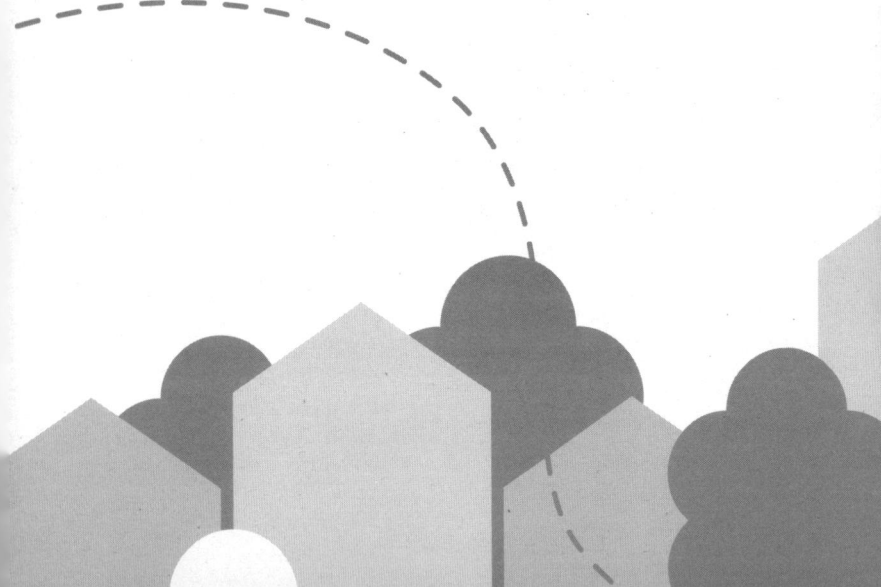

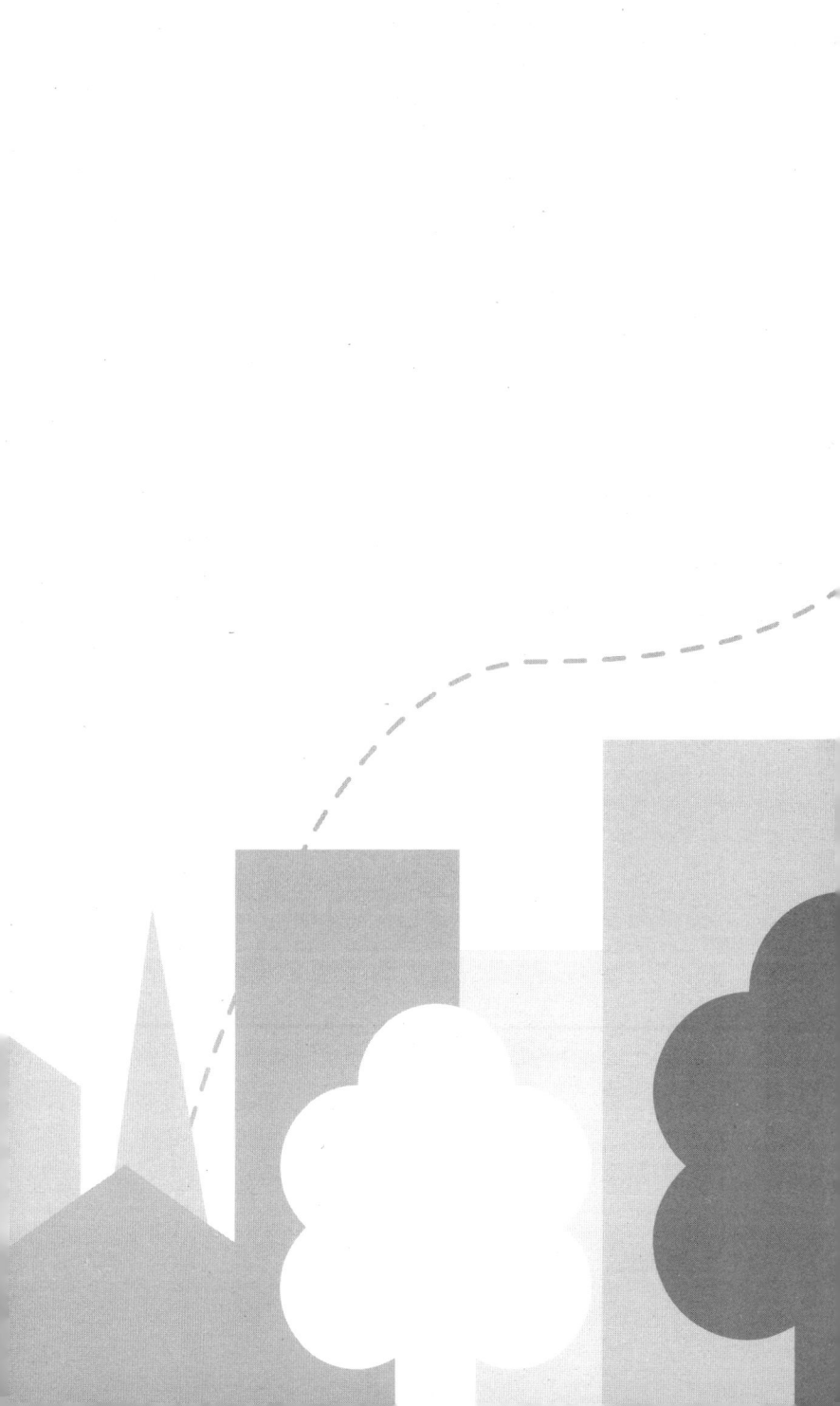

Flatlands

— — — — — — — —

The Bewitching Biology of Space

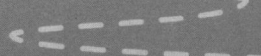

'The flat country – it takes
a hold of you . . . when I strike
the open plains, something
happens. I'm home. I breathe
differently . . .'

WILLA CATHER, INTERVIEW

— — — — — — — —

DEFINITION: Land without hills,
valleys or mountains.

BENEFITS FOR: Feeling confined, trapped or stifled,
excessive self-focus, anxiety, low mood, a need for
clarity and connection.

Noreen Masud's childhood was one of near imprisonment. From her cramped and crowded Lahore home – where friends were banned, where windows were wrapped in chicken wire, where she slept five to a room – an utterly flat landscape, glimpsed through a car window on her drive to school, provided a few moments of daily psychic salvation.

In her memoir, *A Flat Place*, Masud describes these fleeting moments when, on her drive to school, the city suddenly vanished and 'all I could see, stretching out for miles, were huge empty fields'. She loved the greenery and the miracle of 'so much empty land'. But, above all, she loved the flatness.

Masud stored this 'flat place' in her memory. When life became unbearably oppressive, she recalled it and pictured herself moving in ways that were impossible at home – walking, rolling, cartwheeling and 'running . . . faster than was possible, stretching my muscles as hard as they could be stretched'.

"Flat places invite us to live alongside uncertainty"

Later, having fled Pakistan and the grip of her controlling father, Masud realised that the flatness lodged in her mind's eye offered more than a fantasy of space in which to escape. It also reflected aspects of her constrained childhood: 'The field told me . . . that I wasn't mad, that I knew something important . . . and [it] would reflect it back to me.'

Masud – who was plagued by constant ailments and eventually diagnosed with complex post-traumatic stress disorder (CPTSD) – began seeking out the flattest possible places in which to walk. In these 'unyielding, silent' landscapes, Masud learned to live with the complications of her childhood. Flat places, she discovered, propel us into 'a kind of contradiction. Everything . . . lies freely open to us. And yet there seems to be nothing to see.' Instead, they invite us to live alongside uncertainty, to accommodate not knowing into our lives: 'A flat landscape tells me that we can never really know ourselves, let alone anyone or anything other . . . That it was all right to be damaged, hurting, solitary.'[1]

Masud isn't the first walker to fall in love with severely lateral spaces. The artist Georgia O'Keeffe relished the empty expanses of the Texan plains: 'I had nothing but to walk into nowhere and the wide sunset,' she wrote, eulogising the 'wonderful emptiness' and reviving 'nothingness'. Sculptor Barbara Hepworth had a similar response to the flatness of

Norfolk, noting the dominance of birds and exclaiming, 'I feel as though I too have wings on such flat earth.' Meanwhile, the writer Willa Cather – who described her beloved prairies as 'bare as a piece of sheet iron' – saw in flatness 'a kind of erasure of personality', which was as liberating as it was humbling.

"Scientists have identified the sky as one of the greatest sources of awe, wonder, the sublime"

I too once craved emptiness. In my stressed-out thirties I began dreaming of deserts – bolts of blank, bleached-white and clutter-free sand. I grew up among hedged fields, tiny valleys, narrow footpaths, so in spite of my desert fantasies, when I later walked in O'Keeffe's footsteps, I fully expected the plains of Texas to either frighten or bore me.[2] Instead, I found my gaze drawn perpetually up and out to the sky. From the bald, empty Plains, the sky was the largest I'd ever encountered. It surrounded me, it made me feel lightened in some way, shifting how I thought and felt. Little wonder that Masud, Cather and O'Keeffe all wrote of the sudden ability to breathe in these places.

> "Participants reported feeling comforted by the vastness of light, air and space"

As it happens, the experience of walking through sky (which is how it felt to me), and its subsequent effect on our mind and lungs, has a name: skychology. Scientists have identified the sky as one of the greatest sources of awe, wonder, the sublime. Studies now suggest that looking at the sky lifts our mood, reduces physical pain and imbues us with a curious sense of connection. When researcher Paul Conway asked a group of participants to look at the sky at regular intervals each day and then record their experience, many reported immediate improvements in mood. 'In addition to feeling calmer, participants experienced a greater sense of connectedness, a more expansive sense of perspective, and a magnified feeling of being in the moment,' he wrote, adding that 'they felt grounded by the sky.' Conway found that the feeling of connection experienced by participants looking skywards was more marked when participants were alone.

Regularly turning their gaze skywards also gave participants a greater sense of potential and possibility. Instead of feeling overwhelmed or frighteningly diminished, many reported feeling comforted by the vastness of light, air and space. Conway – who also noted participants' predilection for sunsets, sunrises, and top-floor flats – concluded that looking up provided a form of emotional regulation, expressed as an amplified sense of calm, clarity and perspective.[3]

Conway's findings reflected those of a pair of environmental psychologists who, a year earlier, had investigated the preferred views of people living in densely populated cities: the most popular and the most psychically restorative views were those containing the most sky.[4] Sky, it appeared, was as psychologically rejuvenating as the more flaunted green and blue spaces of nature and water.

Skychology is nothing new. For our distant ancestors the sky was a source of guidance, support and spiritual nourishment.

Even a mere 150 years ago, the diarist Beatrix Cresswell wrote in her journal of a longing to go 'Blue-doming', which referred to the Victorian trend for communing with God by looking upwards.[5]

But it would be remiss to think that flatlands affect us merely because of the boundless blue sky they offer. What takes place in the sky is equally significant. In 2023, researcher Alex Smalley published a study examining the impact of fleeting weather conditions on mind and mood. 'The effects of nature on our mental health have been extensively researched,' he wrote, but why had no one investigated the human response to weather? And why, he lamented, was the image of blue sky routinely used to signify happiness?

Smalley had a hunch that non-blue skies were, in fact, infinitely more enthralling and therapeutic than the sunshine-blue skies of holiday brochures. His survey of 2,500 participants proved him right. Sunsets, sunrises, thunderstorms and rainbows prompted the most significant spikes in awe – lifting mood, dampening the inflammation that underlies every chronic disease, and nudging us into heightened feelings of calm, empathy and compassion.*[6] Smalley pointed out that 'getting up a bit earlier for sunrise or timing a walk to catch

---

* Covered in 'Week 44: Seek out the Sublime' in my book 52 *Ways to Walk*.

sunset . . . might unlock small but significant bumps in feelings of beauty and awe, which could, in turn, have positive impacts for mental wellbeing.'[7]

How so? When psychologist Michiel van Elk used fMRI to measure the brain activity of people watching awe-inspiring scenes, he noticed that a collection of brain regions termed the 'default-mode network' quietened down – but only when participants were urged to completely immerse themselves in the scene. Moreover, the more awe-inducing the landscape, the less active the default-mode network became.[8]

Think of the default-mode network as the screen saver that kicks into life when our brain isn't fully engaged. But unlike a static screen saver, this network is actively focused on our self. When we're in default mode, we typically dwell on our past, our future, our identity, our aspirations, frets and fears, our relationships with others. At best, we reflect, plan and make sense of our world. At worst, we self-judge, ruminate and worry. An excessively active default-mode network has been linked to major depression[9] and schizophrenia,[10] while a misconnecting network has been implicated in autism, bipolar disorder and ADHD. The default-mode network was only identified two decades ago, but it's becoming clear that when it's excessively activated, our mental and physical health can suffer. If watching a dramatic sky briefly shuts it down, as van

Elk discovered, that must surely be a good thing.

Dramatic skies aren't the only thing to affect us. The perceived vastness of flat landscapes also plays a part. After reading a series of papers hinting that generous spaces precipitated a less self-focused way of being in the world, a team of Dutch psychologists decided to dig a little deeper. They speculated that spacious landscapes might be particularly suited to promoting selflessness, connectedness and positive mood, while mitigating stress, anxiety and negative mood.

"Open space engenders feelings of selflessness and connectedness"

Their speculations make sense: when we feel ourselves diminished by the vast space we're inhabiting (researchers call this 'the small self'), our sense of being physically bounded falls away. We feel less severed from the world, less disconnected. As a consequence, we might feel more bound both to the landscape and to the people we're with. When the Dutch team then ran a series of experiments in which participants engaged with a variety of virtual landscapes, they found that big space did indeed engender feelings of selflessness and connectedness. In flatlands, participants' self-focus turned outwards with more ease. They felt calmer and more contented. In other words, the more spacious and open the landscape, the easier it is to escape the ruminative prison of our own minds.

After a decade studying the psychological impact of small spaces versus large spaces, psychologist Thomas van Rompay summarised his findings like this:

a)   People in states of high anxiety often benefit from being in generously spaced locations.[11]

b)   We are more likely to share personal information when in spacious places.[12]

c)   Spacious natural landscapes can fuel creative and imaginative thinking.[13]

In an age when much of our time is spent indoors, alongside the smallness and narrowness of pixellated screens, often focusing excessively on our self (our image, identity, plans and goals), walking flatlands with their unlimited panorama of brain-quietening space and sky may be exactly the medicine we need.

There's a final explanation for why flatlands might appeal to so many – and particularly to women. O'Keeffe noted it in her letters when she explained that, although local people warned her from walking alone, she felt safe on the plains. She could see anything coming from miles away, she said, including a change of weather. With nowhere for a predator to hide, flatlands give us a sense of safety and certainty. The vastness gives us a chance to escape or change direction, should we need to, while the flatness means that any forced escape won't be too debilitating, unlike escaping up a mountain, or over a cliff, river or glacier, for example.

It isn't only writers, artists and psychologists who've noticed the remarkable effects of capacious flatness on the human psyche. As mentioned in Chapter 4, the philosopher Gaston Bachelard believed that huge, unfamiliar space was 'the friend of being'. Confronted by its immensity, we humans are able to recognise that 'immensity is within ourselves'.[14] We are cleansed and renewed. We are given hope and possibility. We have space in which to grow and *become*.

notes

Desperate for flatness? Some of the most famously flat places on the planet include the Australian outback, the mudflats of Schleswig-Holstein in Germany, the Bolivian salt flats of Salar de Uyuni (the flattest place in the world), the Everglades in Southern Florida, the Maldive islands, or the Bonneville salt flats of Utah.

In Europe, the Netherlands, Denmark and Lithuania are famously flat.

Closer to home, try (as Masud did) the East Anglian fens (Cambridge is the UK's flattest county, with Lincolnshire not far behind), the mudflats of Morecombe Bay, Newcastle Moor or Orkney in Scotland. Personally, I'm partial to the flatly windswept North Norfolk coast.

Plains are invariably flat, open and spacious – try the UK's Salisbury Plain, New Zealand's Canterbury Plains, Australia's Nullarbor Plain, the Great Plains of Canada and the US, or Hungary's Pannonian Plain.

Beware the wind in flat places: tie up hair and hats, tuck in scarves, avoid billowing skirts. And zip up litter securely.

Overcast days make for dull skies: studies have found that open spaces with exposed sky offered greater physiological restoration on sunny days.[15]

Walk in the aftermath of a storm whenever possible – storms clear away dust and pollutants, leaving clean air, immaculately scoured skies and more vibrant sunrises and sunsets.

Sunsets and sunrises are particularly striking in the presence of abundant mid-to-high clouds, which reflect sunlight to the ground. Meanwhile, very high-altitude clouds – like cirrus or altocumulus clouds – act as a filter for the sun's rays, resulting in glorious hues of tangerine, crimson and scarlet.

Don't be deterred by winter – rainbows are more common at this time of year (in the UK). Winter is also one of the best times to watch sunsets and sunrises, along with late autumn. According to meteorologist Stephen Corfidi, this is because of the cleaner air. Very dry conditions (like deserts) also produce more lustrous sunrises and sunsets, thanks to the smaller amounts of lingering water vapour.

Look out for nacreous clouds – extravagantly colourful, high-altitude clouds often seen at high latitudes.

On summer-night walks (see Chapter 20, 'Nocturne'), look out for rare noctilucent clouds –luminous silvery-blue clouds that float eerily, like ghosts from another world.

Pay attention to the sonic landscape. Sound is muted as it travels, and is absorbed and reflected by trees, buildings and hills. Without these obstacles, we're more likely to hear far-off sounds (which can appear further amplified at night, see Chapter 20, 'Nocturne').

Pack provisions – plains and flatlands can often be surprisingly, bleakly, short of places to eat, drink or shelter.

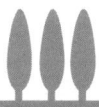

Clifftops

The Miracle of Micro-Climbs

'I trudged on foot along
copper-coloured cliffs . . .
and was . . . elated.'

SIMONE DE BEAUVOIR, *THE PRIME OF LIFE*

— — — — — — — — — —

DEFINITION: An area of land at the top of a cliff.

BENEFITS FOR: The nervous hiker with ambition;
the walker who wants to be alone – but not fully alone;
rebuilding independence, autonomy and respect
for your body.

n 1931, a young Simone de Beauvoir left her home city of Paris and arrived in Marseille, 'sluggish, negative and dejected'.[1] Desperately lonely, suffering from a deficit of ideas, and aware that the man she loved (Jean-Paul Sartre) was both far away and routinely unfaithful, Beauvoir reluctantly settled into her first teaching job.

But Beauvoir disliked the well-heeled 'fat little girls' in her class, and their parents began complaining about her teaching methods. She disliked her fellow teachers too, noting 'that we had nothing in common'. Bereft of friends and family, gripped by envy, disappointment and a yearning for Paris, and with a job and colleagues she loathed, Beauvoir knew she needed a reminder of the joys of life. She also needed to reconstruct herself, to learn 'to be alone'. But how was she to do this?

One day, Beauvoir – who had never hiked – caught a bus to nearby Cassis and began walking over the cliffs. The clifftops were a revelation: when the trail ended ten kilometres later, she was overcome by an urge to do the entire walk all over again. For the next few months Beauvoir spent her free days walking the Calanques – the clifftops south of Marseilles – propelling herself out of her 'emotional, hormonal and metaphysical confusion'. She hiked alone, wearing espadrilles and an old dress, with a basket of buns and bananas balanced on her wrist – to the amusement of other walkers.

Significantly, these walks allowed Beauvoir to begin the slow process of rebuilding muscles that had withered from her long hours of study and a childhood bereft of sport. As she climbed up and down the cliffs, she rid herself of a 'clumsy, gawky' body and simultaneously bolstered her independence and autonomy. Eventually she progressed to more challenging hills and mountains, where she often backpacked for days on end – thanks to the self-belief, inspiration and strength she had discovered on the limestone cliffs of the Calanques. These clifftop walks, she wrote, preserved 'me from boredom, regret and several sorts of depression'.

Much later, as I walked in her footsteps over the cliffs of Cassis and the Calanques, I pondered Beauvoir's choice of landscape. Of all the routes accessible from Marseille, why had she picked clifftops? In truth, it was an inspired decision.

Clifftop walks offer an exhilaration matched only by hills and mountains – and yet they require minimal fitness, kit and navigational skills. Instead of getting lost or bogged down in map-reading (which women were neither trained nor encouraged to do back then), instead of debilitating exhaustion or muscle injury, Beauvoir was able to lose herself in the landscape – forests of windswept, twisted trees on one side, the glistening blue sea on the other. Much later she wrote of the 'self-satisfaction' she derived from these walks, adding, 'I no longer despised myself.'[2]

Clifftop walks require short, repeated up-and-downs – ascents and descents that force our heart to speed up and then slow down. These are not the intimidatingly steep ascents of mountains, nor the rugged, knee-jolting descents of hills. For someone like Beauvoir, wanting to extend herself bit by bit, clifftop walks were an excellent landscape in which to test the capabilities of her own body.

Clifftop routes are also excellent for learning 'to be alone again'. These trails are often popular with other walkers, so we can amble solo but without feeling either abandoned or exposed. We can interact with others without compromising our own solitude.

On a more functional note, walking on an incline is particularly good for the glutes (the muscles in our buttocks), and strong glutes reduce the chance of lower-back pain – making cliff walks and hill walking particularly good for those with sedentary lives. Like many students, Beauvoir had spent hours in libraries and at her desk. We now know that prolonged sitting wreaks havoc with the health of our spine. In the last decade dozens of studies have explored the detrimental physiological effects of prolonged sitting, linking it to error-making, heart disease, high blood pressure, diabetes, osteoporosis, even cancer. In fact, several studies explicitly link excessive sitting to a shorter life.[3]

In 2021, researchers examined the link between prolonged sitting and mood, finding a clear link between lengthy sitting and depression: 'Total and prolonged sitting were associated with a 14 per cent increased odds of . . . depression,' they concluded.[4]

Interestingly, this study found no link between sedentary behaviour and anxiety. But in a later experiment, researchers were surprised to find that although lengthy sitting generated no anxiety if the participants were reading a book, the results changed dramatically when they were hunched over a screen. Students who sat for over two hours with a screen reported rising levels of anxiety,[5] regardless of whether they were relaxing with a film or scrolling on social media. The screen itself seemed to determine whether extended sitting made participants anxious or not. Moreover, the longer they sat with their screens, the greater their levels of anxiety.

How to explain this? The blue light emanating from a screen? The change in seated position demanded by curling over a small screen? Scientists aren't sure, but I think the message is clear: take a screen-free walk.

But let's return to the gently repeating, muscle-building ups and downs that a clifftop amble offers, because the discovery that most astonishes me comes from a 2023 study which tracked over 22,000 people who followed no structured exercise programme – no regular sport, gym membership, Zumba classes or long hikes, for example. Participants were given digital wrist trackers that recorded heart rate, step count and calorie expenditure over the course of a typical week. Seven years later, the researchers compared this data with participants' clinical health records. They found that brief bursts of vigorous activity were linked to a sharply reduced risk for all cancers, but particularly for breast, lung, liver, kidney, colon, endometrial and bowel cancers.

"The landscape itself eases us into a state of health-enhancing breathlessness"

Lead researcher Professor Stamatakis referred to these brief bursts – typically a minute of climbing stairs, walking quickly for a bus, carrying heavy shopping – as 'vigorous intermittent lifestyle physical activities' (catchily abbreviated to VILPA) akin to 'applying high-intensity interval training to your everyday life'. Just 3.5 minutes of VILPA each day was associated with an 18 per cent reduction in total cancer risks, while 4.5 minutes a day was associated with a 21 per cent reduction in risk. These figures rose dramatically for cancers associated with being sedentary: 4.5 minutes a day of 'huff and puff' cut the risk of breast, lung and bowel cancer by a third.[6]

> "Our lungs work harder by breathing faster and deeper to pump extra oxygen round the body"

Few activities provide as many short bursts of 'huff and puff' as clifftop walking, where the landscape itself eases us into a state of health-enhancing breathlessness. To counter the additional resistance of gravity, our lungs work harder by breathing faster and deeper to pump extra oxygen round the body. At the same time, our heart accelerates to increase blood flow to our muscles. Moreover, cliffs (and hills) provide constantly varying inclines, further challenging – in a good way – our heart and lungs. Prof. Stamatakis isn't sure why or how this style of walking reduces our risk of cancer but speculates that it 'leads to rapid improvements in heart and lung fitness, which are linked to lower insulin resistance and lower chronic inflammation', both of which are known risk factors for cancer.

Nor is it just our risk of cancer that is dramatically slashed by 'huff and puff'. Earlier studies have shown that our chances of dying from any cause also drop when our lives include multiple tiny bursts of acceleration.

> ## "Cliff walks are among the most beautiful and interesting of all trails"

And what about our minds? Bathed in a rush of hope molecules (most of which respond enthusiastically to more strenuous movement), our mood climbs too – just like the cliffs we're clambering. Or perhaps all the huffing and puffing simply distracts us, forcing us to tune into our bodies and out of our heads.

notes

Cliff walks are among the most beautiful and interesting of all trails – allowing us to experience many of the benefits of enriched sea air (see Chapter 2, 'Shorelines'), but with the added benefits derived from ascents and descents (see also Chapter 4, 'Rolling Hills' and Chapter 18, 'Mountains').

Clifftops provide us with two simultaneously very different landscapes: on one side the ocean and on the other scrubland, woods, pasture or even the disused remains of maritime industries.[7] Either way, few walks offer the unending variety and distraction of a clifftop walk.

Walking poles can help with speed and balance on both ascents and descents. Studies show that poles help us walk faster but without feeling any more fatigued. As we go downhill, poles take the weight from our knees and make us less likely to fall.

Take binoculars to watch diving birds and sailing ships.

In extreme heat (and wind), shorelines and clifftops can be brutally exposed. Tie up hair, hats and flapping clothes if windy. Take sunscreen: the UV is always higher beside the sea – and that includes clifftops

CHAPTER 9

– and remember sunglasses/hats to avoid the glare of sun on sea.

Like other large expanses of water, the ocean viewed from clifftops provides an abundance of mood-lifting light (see Chapter 10, 'Lakes').

Lakes

- - - - - - -

The Secret Science of Still Water and Light

'A lake is a landscape's most beautiful and expressive feature. It is Earth's eye; looking into which the beholder measures the depth of his own nature.'

HENRY DAVID THOREAU

DEFINITION: A large area of water surrounded by land.

BENEFITS FOR: Inner turmoil, loss, an urgent need for calm.

n 2009, Dr Ali Foxon was working as a climate-change scientist in Switzerland when her world began to fracture, bit by bit.

'My fiancé's mother was diagnosed with aggressive cancer and died five days before our wedding,' she explains. 'Then our son was born prematurely and struggled to sleep. And then my beloved father died suddenly, quite out of the blue.' To make matters worse, Ali was diagnosed with severe endometriosis and told she couldn't have any more children. 'I felt as though I'd been hit by an avalanche. I was emotionally and physically wiped out.' Alone with a small, very awake baby, in a country that wasn't home, Dr Foxon struggled to comprehend the weight of so much grief and loss.

Despite her fatigue, she began taking long walks. 'I was very lonely, with no support network nearby. And I was too shattered and shy to join any local groups,' she told me. 'I knew I was on the verge of depression – it runs in my family – but walking the shores of Lake Geneva was the first step in my recovery. The lake calmed me, but it also inspired me.'

The second step in Dr Foxon's recovery came as she noticed the flash and gleam of sunlight falling first on the lake and then on the emerald feathers of a passing drake: 'I wanted to capture the moment on paper, so I started sketching.' Shortly after, Dr Foxon experienced a lakeside moment of such light-sharpened clarity she felt compelled to make the most reckless, courageous decision of her life. She left her job as a scientist to become an artist.

'Lake Geneva was the perfect place to walk and sketch,' she explains. 'As a hesitant beginner, I welcomed the range of still and slow-moving nature – swans, sleeping ducks, a drifting leaf. Sketching the gentle pace of life on a lake helped me settle my anxious, racing mind.'

Besides, Dr Foxon had a pram to push and a backpack of baby essentials to lug around. 'I was lucky to live near a lake, as I didn't have the energy to venture far, let alone into the mountains. The lake shore was flat and had plenty of benches where I could rest or sketch.'

But it wasn't just the practicalities of lakeside walking that appealed to Dr Foxon. It was also the extra lumens. 'I was instinctively drawn to the light – the sparkling water, the reflections and the vast panorama of pale blue. The light and sense of space soothed my nervous system and brightened my mood,' she explained. 'I could feel myself becoming more resilient by the day.'

I know this inarticulate craving for light. On my morning walks I invariably find myself veering towards the lightest and brightest of spaces. On woodland walks I often seek out the widest and most open of paths, or pause in pools of shimmering opalescent light where the sun streams through the branches of a tree. These aren't decisions I consciously make: I simply follow my body sun-wards.

So why does our biology tug us towards the light? And why is light so important in lifting our mood? Morning light contains an abundance of blue, which helps shut down lingering melatonin left over from the night. According to circadian expert Satchin Panda, melatonin (the hormone that tells our body when to sleep) can linger for an hour after we've woken up, making us feel drowsy, even a little muddle-headed. A shot of bright morning light with its plentiful blue wavelengths – shorter, of higher frequency and carrying more energy – also triggers our body to produce cortisol, a hormone commonly associated with stress. In fact, we need small doses of cortisol to keep us alert, focused and energetic.

This isn't the only reason so many of us are drawn towards the sun. We humans are besotted with light because, as diurnal creatures dependent on our sight, we feel safe when doused in its brilliant rays. Indeed, recent studies[1] show that light also blunts the amygdala, the brain region often referred to as our threat-detection centre or our emotion and fear hub. Put simply, when our amygdala senses something is wrong, it activates our fight-or-flight system, flooding us with the biochemicals necessary for survival. When we're in the grip of chronic stress or anxiety, light quietens our amygdala. And nowhere is as lavishly light as a lake, partly thanks to the sun glitter created when sun hits the surface of clean water. Sun glitter is made up of thousands of tiny glints, each of which is caused by a splinter of sunbeam reflecting at exactly the right angle to send light to our eyes. As breeze or current cause the water to move, so the glitter pattern changes, providing endless light and visual stimulation. Only the ocean produces as much light as a voluminous lake (see Chapter 2).

"People living beside large bodies of water typically feel less stressed"

But bright morning light does more than relieve us of anxiety. New studies show that participants tasked with learning by ear perform better in the presence of blue light than either darkness or orange-hued light. In one study,[2] participants had their brains scanned during a learning task. In the presence of blue light, connections between different pathways in the brain strengthened, improving participants' concentration and memory. Neuroscientists think that our brains have evolved to learn during daylight hours, explaining why other experiments have found that students perform better when classrooms are fitted with blue-rich lights.[3] For Dr Foxon, sketching while on her morning lakeside walk may have accelerated her artistic progress and, therefore, her confidence.

Light has also been linked to mood, with a growing body of evidence suggesting that we need bright light during the day and complete darkness at night (see Chapter 20, 'Nocturne'), rather than the constant low-level and screen-lit illumination that so many of us now live with. A recent study of over 86,000 people found a clear link between increased exposure to sunlight by day and a lower risk of self-harm, anxiety, psychosis, PTSD and major depressive disorder, with those exposed to the brightest light having a 20 per cent lower risk.[4]

How so? The researchers aren't sure, but they suspect that cells at the backs of our eyes, called intrinsically photosensitive retinal ganglion cells, feed information from light photons not only to our primary circadian clock but to two brain regions known for their association with depression (the medial amygdala and the lateral habenula).[5] Perhaps we evolved to feel steadily cheerful when the sun rose – a simple prompt to get up, forage, find water, care for our communities, stay alive.

When Dr Craig McDougall of the University of Stirling investigated the relationship between the mental health of older adults and proximity to large expanses of water, he found that both Scottish lochs and the sea were associated with lower use of antidepressants – but the association was more marked when participants spent time near capacious freshwater lakes. 'Having large amounts of nearby blue space seemed to have a greater impact on antidepressant medication than neighbourhood green space, and lochs stumped the ocean,' he said. Other studies have noted that people living beside large bodies of water typically feel less stressed, but what's interesting is that, when it comes to lakes, size matters. 'The greater the amount of water, the better the local mental health appeared to be, as reflected by the fall in antidepressant prescriptions,' McDougall added.[6]

"When it comes to lakes, size matters"

Meanwhile, studies of animals suggest that a deficit of regular bright light leads to impaired learning, poorer memory and plummeting levels of the biochemicals governing brain plasticity. The authors of two studies of rats incarcerated in conditions of continuous dim light added that 'the behavioural deficits seen in females were more severe than those seen in males'.[7] In other words, males and females respond differently to a lack of bright light. Although we need more research to better understand the impact of light on our brains and bodies, it's becoming increasingly clear that our 'light diet' dramatically affects our physical and mental health.

"Still-water bodies prompted greater feelings of serenity"

And the more time outside the better. When researchers analysed data collected from 500,000 adults, they found that for each additional hour spent in outdoor light, participants experienced a corresponding fall in their risk of developing depression. To boot, the more time participants spent in natural light, the less they used antidepressants and the happier they felt.[8] More recently, Chinese researchers investigating the restorative properties of Hangzhou lake pinpointed sunny days as those which produced the highest feel-good factor among lakeside walkers.[9]

But do we really prefer still fresh water to moving fresh water? Well, yes, it appears that many of us do. When researchers asked a group of Scottish participants to record their mood, emotions and responses to all types of water using daily diaries, they were surprised to find that still-water bodies, such as lakes and reservoirs, prompted greater feelings of serenity than running water like rivers and streams.[10]

So, other than the amplified sense of light, what is it about the stillness of water that makes us feel so rejuvenated? Some scientists have noted the meditative and reflective qualities of still water, but researcher Megan Grace, who led the study above, thinks that the sense of lakeside space may play a part. She told me that 'participants particularly enjoyed the openness of lake spaces and found them very relaxing compared to more enclosed walks along river paths'.[11]

"Water encourages us to relax"

Dr Foxon agrees. 'Lakes are wonderfully calm and consistent,' she says. 'Much as I love the sea, I tend to keep a cautious eye on the waves and tide, especially with a baby. It was far easier to walk, sketch and fully relax on the shores of Lake Geneva.' And herein lies another truth of still water: free from fretting about rising tides, wayward currents, jellyfish, or freak waves, we feel safe.

For blue-space researcher Dr Catherine Kelly, all water is good: 'Being in or next to water reduces our blood pressure, slows our breathing and allows our parasympathetic nervous system to do its job. This is our "rest, repair and repose" system and it's vital for effective brain function and a strong immune system. Water encourages us to relax ... Being in and near water reduces the stress hormones cortisol and adrenaline that can make us feel unwell.'[12]

"Being in and near water reduces the stress hormones cortisol and adrenaline"

But Dr Kelly also acknowledges the remarkable power of *still* water. 'Reflected light links the visual environment to human feelings,' she told me. 'Lake water has texture that easily sparkles, reflects or ripples with the wind, evoking what psychologists call "soft fascination", effortless attention accompanied by aesthetic pleasure. Our brain switches off from our daily worries.'[13]

Anyone unconvinced that water holds a profoundly affective grip on the human psyche should take heed of a 2023 survey where behavioural scientists compared the mindset of people living in watery places with the mindset of those inhabiting water-deprived areas. They found marked differences, explaining that inhabitants of dry landscapes were more 'cautious and future-oriented' and spent more time planning and thinking ahead, while inhabitants of water-rich regions were more likely to live in the moment and have fun. Being without water, said the researchers, 'prompts a general mindset of thrift and long-term thinking', adding that evolution has wired us to react unequivocally to the promise of abundant water and to the threat of water scarcity.[14]

Just make sure the water you're hiking beside is clean. No one wants to gaze at floating plastic bottles and crisp packets. For some of the clearest, cleanest water, head for Scottish lochs, Finnish lakes and Alpine tarns. Earth's eye in every way.

notes

How long? Within three minutes of lake-gazing, our stress levels fall dramatically, according to researchers in Hong Kong who used EEG to monitor the brainwaves of people water-watching.[15]

Don't restrict your walks to sunny days. A 2023 study found that 'spaces with calm water' were more emotionally restorative on cloudy days than on sunny days.[16]

Take a sketch book and pencil. Dr Foxon believes that drawing can help pull us out of our own heads. She urges sketchers to focus on the observation, not the artwork.

Much like sketching, diary keeping can be therapeutic. Studies show that diarists found writing about their experiences of lake-walking encouraged them to be more reflective, more actively immersed in the life of the lake. Take a notebook and record how the lake makes you feel.

The amount of light reflected from the surface of a lake depends on several factors, including its surface area, clarity and depth (the larger, clearer and shallower the better), as well as the angle of the sun (the lower the better) and the movement of the water. For energy and mood-boosting blue-wave light, take your lakeside walk in the morning.

Sun glitter is also spectacular at the end of the day when light beams pass through miles of atmosphere, scattering away most of the blue light and creating glitter in shades of crimson, pink, amber and gold – and telling our body that it's time to wind down.[17] Moonlight on still water creates its own 'moon glitter' (see Chapter 20, 'Nocturne') and is well worth seeking out for its eerily mysterious elegance.

Sun is as good for our heart (and our fertility!) as our minds: 2024 studies have linked higher exposure to natural light with lower rates of heart failure[18] and to greater fertility in older women[19] – for reasons that appear to go beyond vitamin D. Some researchers speculate that the deep violet and infrared light blocked by glass (including eyewear) may have overlooked benefits for vision, germ control and even brain health..

Lakes are often popular wild-swimming spots. Again, there's evidence that wild swimming can also help us maintain our equilibrium, triggering the body to produce a torrent of feel-good, vigour-inducing biochemicals, including dopamine and norepinephrine. Pack a towel and take a dip.

As optics scientist Joseph Shaw said, 'Beautiful light shows can be seen by anyone with the attention to notice . . . you can either casually notice these patterns or spend hours examining them in detail . . . there is much to be learned and much to be appreciated about nature by watching light glittering on water.'[20] And nowhere is better for a light show than a lake.

Ghostlands

Biochemical Bonding on
Disused Railway Lines

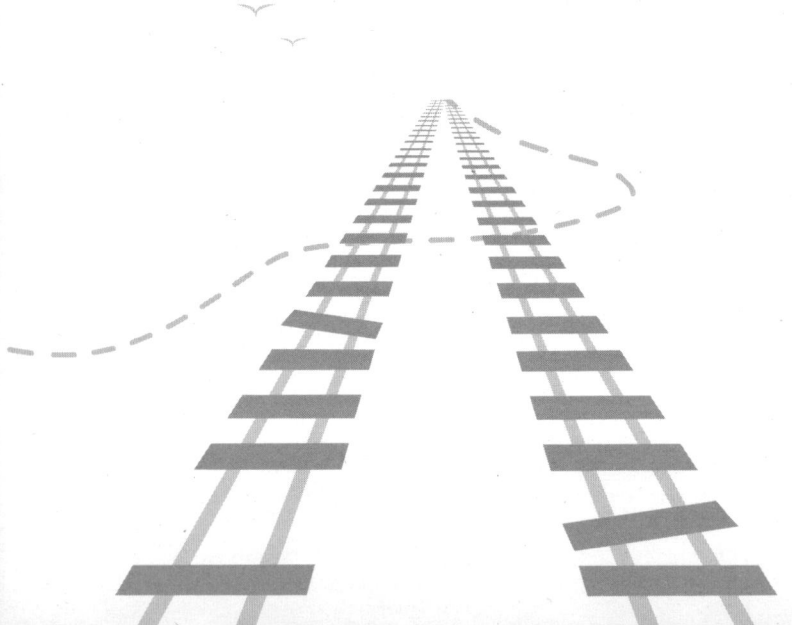

'You see the bridges, viaducts, tunnels, cuttings and embankments. You might come across the remains of an old signal, old mile posts or the gradient posts with arms pointing up or down to show the gradient . . . if you need something gentle to get started, railway lines are ideal.'

JEFF VINTER, *VINTER'S RAILWAY GAZETTEER*[1]

— — — — — — — —

DEFINITION: A railway line no longer used to carry trains.

BENEFITS FOR: Families and friends wanting to boost or repair their bonds; those in need of creative and imaginative fuel; the grieving and bereaved; anyone frustrated at today's technological age; parents feeling oppressed by lack of space.

Ask any writer for their favourite walk and, chances are, they'll give you the name of a disused or abandoned railway line. *Trainspotting* author Irvine Walsh says his favourite walk when in his home city of Edinburgh is the disused railway line to Portobello Beach. Renowned writer Hunter Davies was so enamoured of railway walks, he wrote a book about them. Meanwhile, the bestselling author Emma Healey turns routinely to the Lakenham Way in Norfolk when in need of inspiration.

What is it about disused railway lines that make them so appealing to writers? Abandoned railway lines, says Healey, are 'in-between places' – neither completely rural nor strictly urban. She describes them as 'atmospheric and inspiring', tracks that 'feel like writing itself'.[2] I experienced something similar in remote rural France, when I discovered that the residency where I was staying backed onto 76 km of old disused railway line, known as a *voie verte*. As I walked it daily, my book effortlessly unfurled, like the track ahead of me. The line was deserted, so I often wrote 'aloud', recording snippets into my phone.

And yet, despite the thousands and thousands of secret, forgotten tracks all over the world, many of us avoid these landscapes. We prefer a circular walk, or a walk with more to see and do. With our innate preference for views, we head for the hills and mountains. With our hardwired love of water, we make a beeline for lakes, rivers, canals and coast. For many of us, railway tracks just don't feature on our list of favourite places to walk.

But the science suggests we may have been too hasty in writing off railway trails. When we amble a railway track, changes often take place deep within our brains, allowing us to return home with new ideas. We already know that walking and nature spark more imaginative thinking. A 2021 article in *Harvard Business Review* listed both walking and 'green space' as two of the four best prompts for creative thinking.[3] But a disused railway line goes further.

"These are often the quietest and most uniform of walks"

Like a canal towpath, a disused railway line requires no map-reading or navigation whatsoever. We simply step onto the track and follow it, for as long as we need. Most tracks start in urban areas (often close to existing train stations), meaning we can easily get there without a car. More importantly, as we walk a railway line, we can completely switch off. Knowing we won't get lost, that we don't need to navigate or map-read, that we need do nothing but walk, frees our brain of any drop of the chemicals now thought to inhibit imaginative thought (see Chapter 13, 'Canal Towpaths').

In fact, a railway line might be more conducive to deep imaginative work than a towpath because it usually offers fewer distractions. For those of us wanting as little mental interruption as possible, a disused railway line can pip all landscapes: these are often the quietest and most uniform of walks.

> "Walking these newly lost landscapes can be profoundly affecting"

But railway lines have more to offer imaginatively than ease of navigation and lack of distraction. While canals are still used by longboats and barges, even if only for recreational purposes, disused railway lines have become utterly disconnected from their original raison d'etre. These are ghost trails, landscapes severed from their own past. And yet, as we walk them, we encounter regular reminders of their very recent history – from abandoned stations to tunnels, signal boxes, bridges, even sections of old track. When we walk a railway line we are imaginatively thrown back, not to the distant, long-gone past (see Chapter 12, 'Therapeutic Landscapes'), but to the lives of our grandparents and great-grandparents. Here the past is so close we can sense its almost pulsing presence.

Walking these newly lost landscapes can be profoundly affecting. Railway lines once connected ports and quarries, cities and coal mines, towns and mills, reminding us of an industrial age that dramatically shaped our current world. But railways also carried families to unknown places – to the seaside, to the mountains, to distant relatives – for the very first time. With the railway came the concept of holidays and the notion of travel for adventure, opportunity or escape. In the world wars of the last century, trains changed the face of warfare, carrying thousands of soldiers across Europe, Africa and Asia.

With the slightest of imaginative effort, we can hear the whistle of a freight train loaded with coal or quarry stone. We can catch the excited cries of children bound for the seaside, the hiss of steam, the clatter and rattle of the tracks. Disused railways are ghost places, reminding us of the brevity of man-made things, of the transience of technologies, of how loss and change have always shaped our lives and our landscapes. Here we can reconstruct the world of a generation back. But we can also examine what has come and gone in our own lives and how we too have been shaped by change and loss. Alone on a railway path, amid hand-dug cuttings, laboriously laid tracks and intricately designed bridges, we can reflect on the ephemerality of all that we build, reminding ourselves that we have always lived amid uncertainty – and survived, even thrived.

Once-bustling places of speed, progress and modernity, disused railway lines remind us that earthly things are not always as they seem. When we walk a railway line, our imaginations slowly turning, we understand that transformation is a complicated and nuanced thing, that there is beauty and soul in absence, that fester and decay are merely part of the tapestry of life. In the cathartic mode of walking induced by a ghostscape, we see too that fester and decay are – in fact – landscapes of hope. Today's abandoned lines have become quivering corridors of wildlife, much of it unusual or rare.

"Many disused railway lines are now home to rare plants, insects, mammals and birds"

How has this happened? Partly, of course, because these places have been left to themselves, free from people and pesticides. More intriguingly, though, we may need to pay tribute to their cuttings, also known as embankments – the steep sides dug (often by hand) to keep railway lines flat. As I walked the *voie verte*, I grew to love the cuttings – which made me feel safely unexposed and comfortingly contained, a pair of arms that kept me in the right place. Later, I discovered that cuttings were one of the idiosyncrasies of this landscape, enabling wildlife to proliferate.

Cuttings provide both sunny south-facing slopes and sheltered north-facing banks, allowing for more diverse flowers, trees and grasses. With this come more diverse insects, mosses and fungi, bringing a greater number of birds and small mammals. Moreover, the length of many old tracks has made them valuable corridors, meaning mammals are less likely to become roadkill. In fact, many disused railway lines are now home to rare plants, insects, mammals and birds.

CHAPTER 11

"No landscape is as delightfully democratic as a railway path"

But these are not the only gifts of a railway ghostscape, and the French *voie verte* was not my first experience of a rail trail. As a mother of young children, a fourteen-mile line through Sussex called the Cuckoo Trail had been one of my favourite, sanity-saving routes. Here I spent many days with my children and labrador dog, enjoying a flat, even scape where the eldest could cycle, the next down could pretend to be a train, the toddler could totter, the baby could be pushed in his pram, the dog could be safely released from her lead and my ageing parents-in-law could shuffle unhurriedly beside us. For a new parent, a railway line carries none of the anxiety that accompanies a canal towpath, a road or a clifftop: without water, traffic or precipices, we can wholly relax. No landscape is as delightfully democratic as a railway path.

On the Cuckoo Trail, I also discovered that disused railway lines were surprisingly and beautifully bonding. After yomping up and down, my family and I often returned home with a replenished intimacy, which I assumed was the result of fresh air, greenery and movement.

I was right – to a point. But now science suggests that a hormone and neurotransmitter called oxytocin may have played a part in our 'railway-track bonding'. Oxytocin (often called the love hormone) was discovered over a century ago, when it was found to trigger labour pains.

But back in the 1970s, East German scientists exploring biochemical opportunities for furthering their Olympic prowess noticed that blood concentrations of oxytocin increased in response to physical and mental exertion – for instance, marathon runners and chess players produced more oxytocin as they strove, both physically (the runners) and cognitively (the chess players). Oxytocin – it appeared – was more than just a promoter of uterine contractions and breast-milk let-down.

Since then, scientists have discovered that oxytocin is nuanced and complex, interacting with multiple other traits and factors both biological and circumstantial – and frequently nothing to do with reproduction. We know, for example, that oxytocin dilates our arteries, helping blood, oxygen and nutrients swiftly reach our heart. It appears to protect against ageing and inflammation, with some researchers pondering whether raised levels of oxytocin could protect the brain from cognitive degeneration.

In the meantime, its ability to curb hunger pangs means

oxytocin is being explored as a weight-loss medicine, while its pain-relieving features suggest that it could have a future role in pain relief.[4] Most intriguingly of all, oxytocin is being investigated for its anti-anxiety and anti-depressant possibilities. The more oxytocin tumbling through our veins, the calmer and more cheerful we are. As one team of researchers put it, 'the oxytocin system may have the capacity to alleviate detrimental physiological and mental stress reactions'.[5]

And to top it all, oxytocin is also being investigated as a neurohormone that enhances creativity.

So how do we encourage our bodies to produce more oxytocin? And how can a walk along a railway line aid this process?

Like the biochemicals mentioned in the Introduction, oxytocin is now deemed an exerkine, a hope molecule activated by movement. Studies show that ten to fifteen minutes of brisk movement raised circulating levels of oxytocin (in men and women) by two and a half times.[6] As with most hope molecules, our walk must be heart-pumping – although future research may be able to shed more light on just how fast we need to be moving.

But it's not just *how* we walk: *where* we walk can also boost oxytocin levels. In places where we feel safe, calm and less fearful, we typically produce more oxytocin. 'Areas that are perceived as familiar and attractive [as well as safe and calm] stimulate oxytocin release, which in turn exerts powerful anti-stress effects,' wrote researchers in a 2021 paper exploring the links between oxytocin and being in nature.[7]

Curiously, oxytocin increases when our movements are synchronised with those of people we like, explaining why walking or running alongside family and friends can be an oddly restorative and bonding experience. If we stop and hug one of our teammates for around twenty seconds, our levels of oxytocin increase yet again. Likewise, petting our dog also releases oxytocin (in both us and the dog, according to the latest experiments[8]).

As a new mother I was probably already swimming in a sea of oxytocin. The railway line, however, was wide enough that we could walk side by side holding hands – another action that produces oxytocin. Without traffic or water to contend with, we could run, jump and shimmy. We often sang (another oxytocin generator), and we regularly paused to stroke passing dogs.

Oxytocin is currently thought of as a person- (or pet-) prompted chemical, but it's also a chemical of connection. I have a sneaking suspicion that future researchers will discover that certain places – those we fall upon as if they were old friends – might also prompt a surge of oxytocin. Professor Bertram Opitz hinted as much in his study of place for the

National Trust, writing, 'the brain treats meaningful places very differently to everyday places . . . [they] generate a strong emotional response'. Opitz linked this sort of connection to 'higher levels of wellbeing . . . greater happiness, life satisfaction and feeling life is worthwhile'.[9]

notes

Europe – and much of the world – is criss-crossed by thousands of miles of forgotten or disused railway track (4,000 miles in the UK and considerably more in France, Austria, Italy and Germany). Many – but not all – of these have been transformed into magnificent walking and cycling routes, replete with viaducts, tunnels and wildlife-rich cuttings. Search online or buy a guidebook – and start exploring.

As you walk, try and muster images of your ancestors using railways. I think of my grandfather returning from the war, my grandmother waiting for him at the station. If your imaginings precipitate a feeling of empathy, all the better: studies suggest that when we feel empathy, we produce oxytocin.[10]

Sing as you walk with family or friends. Singing with others is another proven way of making more oxytocin, with studies showing that choirs have more circulating oxytocin than solo singers.[11]

Hold hands, wrap your arms around children, friends, partners –

touch (particularly when skin to skin) also promotes the release of oxytocin.

Pause to pat and cuddle (friendly) dogs. Stroking animals is an instant source of oxytocin.

The vitamin D made by sunshine is thought to help synthesise oxytocin, so choose a sunny day and roll up your sleeves.

Talk as you walk – intimate conversations can generate oxytocin. Friendly smiles and voices from strangers have also been found to trigger its release, so greet and smile at passers-by.[12]

To spot some of the smaller insects and lichens that love a cutting, take a loupe – a tiny magnifying glass (much loved by children) that can be used to examine moss, mushrooms, moths and maggots!

Reconditioned railway lines are not just for the country. New York's High Line is one of my favourite walks, as is Paris's Promenade Plantée (or Coulée Verte) and London's Parkland Walk, where the old train tunnels have been transformed into bat caves.

Like the idea of exploring more ghostlands on foot? Seek out sunken or abandoned villages, decommissioned nuclear-power stations, forgotten factories, churches and hospitals by visiting sites like urbexhub.com, a cornucopia of images featuring decaying buildings from across the globe. Or head for the Durham Heritage Path, one of my favourite ghostland trails.

Therapeutic Landscapes

The Mysterious Power of Sacred Places

'One feels [in Delphi] a gathered silence as if through the centuries the stones and monuments had drawn into themselves, and now held forever, all the aspirations and questioning, the deepest desires and holiest thoughts of humanity.'

CLARA VYVYAN, *TEMPLES AND FLOWERS: A JOURNEY TO GREECE*

DEFINITION: A space or place with an enduring reputation for achieving physical, mental and spiritual healing.

BENEFITS FOR: Dread of uncertainty, a longing for mystery and magic, an anxious beating heart, fear of death.

When travel writer Jini Reddy began yearning for more magic and mystery in her life, she decided to go looking for it in the many landscapes of Britain. She wanted to experience 'the land . . . in a way that went beyond the ordinary.' Reddy, who had lost both her father and her sister, longed to feel 'more porous . . . a bit Other and a bit mystical even,' she recalled in her memoir, *Wanderland: A Search for Magic in the Landscape.*

'I felt invisible,' she explained, 'I was becoming ill and needy with the desire to be heard.' Reddy knew her sanity was at stake, and the only remedy was to seek out a 'thin' world she obscurely sensed, 'a world that co-exists with the visible one, a world of signs and portents . . . of communion'. Driven by her own 'intimate experience of Otherness' (British by birth, Indian by descent, Canadian by upbringing, South African via her parents' birthplace), Reddy set out to explore some of Britain's more esoteric, magical and spiritual places, from secret healing springs to forgotten land temples and hidden labyrinths.

Each of Reddy's journeys began with a vague, baffled hope. But at the end, she felt profoundly changed, 'as though my DNA has been altered', she wrote, and 'as sharp and clear-headed and rested and full as it is humanly possible to feel. You move through loneliness and disconnection and you get to this, if you're lucky.'

But was it luck? Or was something else at play? The landscapes Reddy walked often had historic reputations as sites of healing. For centuries, these places were walked to and from in an invisible continuity of hope – men wanting cures, women wanting babies, everyone wanting inner resolution or physical rejuvenation. Today, few of us attribute healing qualities to a hidden spring or a circle of standing stones. But perhaps, like Reddy, we should gently question our modern scepticism.

Back in the 1990s, mathematician-turned-social geographer Dr Wil Gesler began pondering the intersection of place, culture and history – a sort of geography of wellbeing. Having studied three traditional places of healing (Lourdes in France, Bath in the UK and Epidaurus in Greece), he coined the term 'therapeutic landscapes' to describe particular settings with an enduring reputation for achieving physical, mental and spiritual healing.

Today the concept of a therapeutic landscape has been extended to cover anywhere associated with recovery – from holy wells and sacred springs to hospitals, spas and the ancestral sites of indigenous peoples. Curiously, the healing powers of some of these places have since been confirmed by scientists and researchers.

The best-tested therapeutic landscape is the healing spring of Lourdes where, in 1858, a young Bernadette

Soubirous encountered the Virgin Mary in a series of visions. Since then, millions of visitors and pilgrims have arrived in search of better health. Many claimed to have been miraculously cured. In 1883, a medical bureau was established at Lourdes to investigate, certify and record 'miracle cures'. According to bureau records, at least a hundred cures took place every year until 1914, after which the number of reported cures steadily declined.[1]

But it wasn't until 2012 that a team of scientists began scrutinising these records. What they found intrigued and surprised them: many of the cures appeared genuine and enduring. 'Uncanny and weird, the cures are currently beyond our ken but still impressive and incredibly effective,'[2] they noted, adding that 'the Lourdes phenomenon, extraordinary in many respects, still awaits scientific explanation'.

The researchers speculated that much of the healing was 'part of a neuropsychiatric phenomenon ... We surmise that autosuggestion and the placebo effect played a role in a number of ... cures.' They noted that at Lourdes (as at other healing sites) there was a high level of 'anticipation and hope, belief and confidence, fervor and awe, meditation and exaltation', all of which compounded 'the spiritual atmosphere of the place'.

A more recent study of Lourdes pilgrims found that almost half reported a transcendent experience: some felt they had 'communicated with a divine presence, while others reported a powerful experience of something intangible and otherworldly'.[3]

"Using our minds, we kindle a physiological healing response"

Studies of Scottish shrines known for their healing powers have also revealed a solace and divinity sensed by those in their presence.[4] Sacred landscapes in Quebec, China, Indonesia, India and Nepal have since been subjected to the rigours of science, with researchers invariably and mysteriously finding 'significant physical and mental health benefits'. As one researcher put it, sacred sites 'have evolved and grown over millennia to become critical sociocultural phenomena'. In other words, it's the knowing, imagining and believing that propel these sites into places of personal transformation.[5]

We underestimate the placebo effect at our peril. The well-documented healing effects of placebos come from us – from our thoughts, beliefs and expectations. Using our minds, we kindle a physiological healing response. And yet studies show that placebo effects can be amplified by those – and that – surrounding us. For example, placebo pills work more effectively when given by doctors that we like and trust.[6]

"The majesty of a place can magnify the feelings of hope we bring to it"

Work done by Stanford University's Mind & Body Lab has consistently found that how we think shapes our mental and physical health. Researchers here believe that 'placebo effects are not mysterious, unexplainable forces, but rather products of psychological and contextual factors.' Their work explores the powerful effects of mindsets, that how and what we think can change us emotionally, psychologically and physiologically. Which is to say, that if we walk a landscape and believe it to be healing, we may – quite possibly – find ourselves healed. As researcher Esther Sternberg reminds us in her account of healing landscapes, 'the belief that something has the capacity to heal is extremely powerful'.[7]

"Places with symbolic meaning have the potential to heal"

Meanwhile, researchers studying pilgrims on the Camino de Santiago (the Way of St James) concluded that the variety of landscape also plays a very significant role in the amplified sense of wellbeing experienced by walkers. The endlessly changing shades, textures and sounds, the awakening of physical senses – these too appeared to heighten the experience, often giving it a 'transcendent' quality.[8] It appears that the majesty of a place can magnify the feelings of hope we bring to it – much as kindly, trusted doctors imbued a placebo pill with greater efficacy in the experiments carried out at Stanford's Mind & Body Lab.

Since then, other studies have come to similar conclusions: that places with symbolic meaning have the potential to heal. A study carried out at a non-denominational spiritual retreat in Michigan, America, revealed a marked increase in hope, known to play a mitigating role in both depression and heart disease.[9] Researchers studying healing sites in Scotland[10] and at Stonehenge have noticed things 'bordering on the realm of the uncanny'. When Dr Claire Nolan interviewed people who regularly walk at Stonehenge, several spoke of 'a tangible special "feeling" in the landscape.'[11]

Many said the stones and the landscape rooted them in an existential way, encouraging them to think more deeply about time, permanence, continuity and tradition. Being there made them feel acutely connected – to the past, the Earth and the cosmos. Some described the Stonehenge and Avebury landscapes as 'essential to their mental wellbeing'. Others spoke of 'peace', 'awe' and 'connectedness'. Nolan noted that the standing stones often provided a sense of security: this was somewhere for reflection, free from the stresses of modern life.

"These landscapes nourish our minds and souls"

'Participants often described feeling as if they are an actual, living part of the landscape and its history,' she told me. 'Some described it as being emotionally held and supported. I've no doubt that walking among prehistoric remains gives many people a greater appreciation of their place in time, the world and the cosmos. It puts their lives into perspective, helping them find greater meaning.'[12] Nolan ended her study with an impassioned plea for a better understanding of how such places nourish our minds and souls.

So how does this 'nourishing' work? Landscapes of spiritual significance – Reddy's 'thin' places – allow us to experience mystery, the unknown and the magical. Here, mind, body and spirit briefly reconnect. For a few moments, we live alongside uncertainty, the unfathomable. To feel at ease with the unknown, however fleetingly, calms us, helping us shunt aside stress and anxiety.

This matters: very recent research suggests that mental stress and our physical health may be more intimately bound up than we thought. Researchers at America's Salk Institute have discovered that the biochemicals produced under stress (and let's be clear, little is more stressful to we humans than uncertainty) dramatically impede the work of vital immune cells called T-cells, a type of white blood cell known for countering infections and fighting cancer. After investigating T-cells in human tissue, researchers were surprised to find that a surfeit of noradrenaline (produced as a result of psychological stress) caused T-cells to abandon the tumours and pathogens they'd been battling, and race to form a cluster around the circulating stress hormones.

When the researchers used beta blockers to dampen the

production of stress hormones, the renegade T-cells started working normally again. Stress hormones, it appears, can stop our immune cells functioning, leaving us dangerously exposed. Countering stress – whether that's via beta blockers or walking through ancient standing stones – could result in more resilient T-cells, leaving us stronger and healthier.[13] All of which is to say, landscapes wherein we surrender willingly to the (often anxiety-inducing) unknown offer an incomparable therapeutic balm.[14]

Today, even scientists devoted to the empirical, to evidence, acknowledge that Homo sapiens may be hardwired for transcendent experiences, that we may even need them. According to physicist Alan Lightman,[15] spiritual experiences are as necessary as food or water. 'Everything is made out of atoms and molecules and nothing more . . . spiritual experience can arise from atoms and molecules [and yet] some of these experiences . . . cannot be fully understood in [these] terms.'

Today, having a sense of spirituality has been repeatedly shown to play an important part in resilience, grit and hope. Studies of migrants, refugees and asylum seekers have found that those who see themselves as 'spiritual' are more likely to recover from trauma,[16] while emergency nurses self-reporting as 'spiritual' were less likely to suffer burnout.[17] A survey of Swiss heart-attack patients found that spirituality was significantly associated with less depression,[18] and a study of people caring for cancer patients concluded that spirituality is 'a significant resource for coping with caregiving challenges'. In other words, a sense of spirituality (whether religious or not) seems to help us weather the ups and downs of life.

notes

Seek out places once deemed 'spiritually healing': wells, holy/sacred springs, river sources/mouths and confluences. Traditionally, walkers either immersed themselves in, or drank from, these water sources.

Use a reputable filter – like Grayl or MSR – before drinking holy water and only bathe if it's safe to do so (take a micro towel and slip in naked, as the indomitable Reddy does).

The British Pilgrimage Trust includes ancient trees (particularly yew trees), caves and hermitages, churches, chapels, cathedrals and temples, holy hills and ruins, and tumuli (from long barrows to stone circles) in its list of potentially healing places. See britishpilgrimage.org/holy-places

Many pilgrim routes begin, traverse and end in therapeutic landscapes (see Chapter 17, 'Distance Trails and Pilgrim Routes'). Alternatively, use Ordnance Survey maps to locate wells, labyrinths, tumuli, churches and springs.

Even very old vineyards have been shown to have therapeutic potential, once their symbolic meanings, traditions and histories have been shared.[19] Knowing the stories underlying therapeutic locations is vital, so do your homework in advance or take a guided walk with an expert.

Equally, going guideless brings its own benefits. In 'thin' landscapes, we can let the land guide us, says Reddy, who sometimes went map-less, following her senses and inclinations instead.

Some people believe these places possess potent energy fields that affect our vitality. Others think that past ancestral activities (be they miracle cures or movement) can be sensed as mysteriously lingering energies.[20] Me? I think anything that lights up our imagination, moving us closer to the pulse of life (whether backed by data or not), deserves exploring.

Still not convinced? Check out the work of five Dutch researchers who, in 2023, investigated miracle cures that had been 'rigorously' assessed and confirmed by the Amsterdam University Medical Centre. These cures, they concluded, were both remarkable and inexplicable.[21]

For something more esoteric, look into astro-archaeology and the work of Katharine Maltwood, who linked ancient landscapes to the sun, stars and moon. Alternatively, take a look at the history of ley lines (search online or see Week 21 of my book *52 Ways to Walk*).

How to feel more hopeful? 'A brisk walk,' suggests Harvard Health,[22] alongside feelings of gratitude (see also Chapter 5, 'Cemeteries'). See Introduction for why walking releases hope molecules.

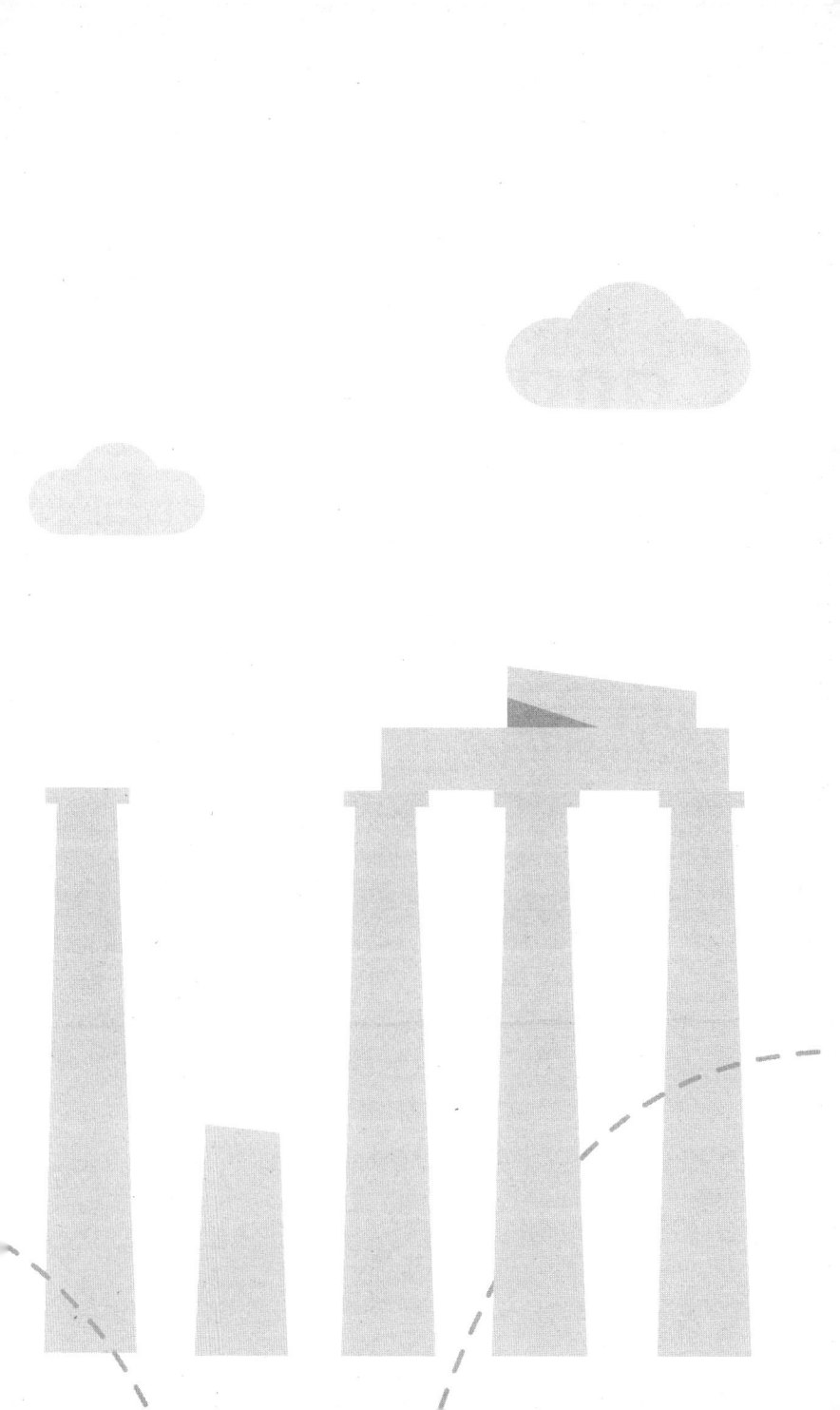

Canal Towpaths

Nourish Your Creativity

'Ask of it – water, help me rise
And water says I will.'

JO BELL, CANAL LAUREATE 2013–15, 'LIFTED'

DEFINITION: A canal is an artificial waterway
constructed to allow the passage of boats or ships inland,
or to convey water for irrigation; a towpath is a path
beside a canal, originally used by horses towing barges.

BENEFITS FOR: Writer's block; episodes of creative
blockage; the times when answers and solutions elude
us; when life feels too hurried; when we need rest.

F or over a decade now, the (British) Canal & River Trust has worked with the Poetry Society, offering an annual place to a Canal Laureate. Walk the towpath of any UK canal and you may well pass a poet reciting their own freshly minted words. The project – called 'Waterlines' – has generated dozens of poems, both from its many Canal Laureates and from those who, having walked the towpaths, feel compelled to create their own verse. 'These 2,000 miles of water,' wrote Canal Laureate Roy McFarlane in 2023, are 'corridors to another world, creating and conjuring . . .'[1]

So what is it about the towpath of a canal that sparks the imagination of so many poets, enabling them to create and conjure?

Unlike any other landscape, canals and their towpaths operate in a liminal in-between place – neither completely natural nor completely man-made, neither all water nor earth, neither strictly rural nor strictly urban. In their melding of brick, water and path with wildlife and wilderness, and as aquatic arteries linking cities with countryside, canals and their towpaths form a uniquely hybrid walking landscape that simultaneously soothes and inspires. Ask any Canal Laureate and they will tell you that canals exist in a fascinating intersection of past and present, of urban and rural, of artificial and wild . . . a waterscape like no other. And one that continuously piques and intrigues, offering tantalising glimpses of long-lost lives while herons unfold their wings from the bank. No other landscape offers this beguiling blend of industry, history, architecture, water and wildlife, green space and blue space, peace and people.

It's not just poets who are waking up to the imaginative promise of canals. A study of over 2,000 office workers, conducted by Glasgow Caledonian University, found those working in offices overlooking docks and canals felt more creative. A third of respondents claimed to not only feel more creative but to be more productive.[2]

Both poets and office workers are right. Canals carry all the joy of water at its most alluring (glimmering light, enticing reflections, fractal ripples, abundant wildlife, bobbing boats). The things that frighten us about water are rarely found in canals – no threat of enormous waves, no current to drag us under, no tide to cut off our path.* Alongside a canal, even our age-old fears of untamed water fade away: this is domesticated water. More poodle than panther, more labrador than leopard.

But why does this make walking a towpath so conducive to creativity? The answer might lie in the unusual combination of absent stress hormones with the linear certitude of a canal.

---

* Far fewer people drown in canals than in sea, lake or river water.

Neuroscientists have recently been exploring the brain mechanisms that contribute to the looser, more connected thinking that appears to generate original ideas and innovative ways of seeing. American neurologist Kenneth Heilman thinks inventiveness comes from 'associative and convergent thinking', which happens when different brain circuits meet and meld.[3] He argues that the hormone epinephrine (the brain's version of adrenaline), blocks 'associative and convergent' thinking by carefully restricting each neuronal circuit to its own zone.

Think of the brain as a cluster of circuits, much like a palette of paints, with each colour in its own tray. For new colours to emerge from our 'palette' we need a splash of water enabling them to spill out, mingle, blend. In the presence of epinephrine (produced by our adrenal glands and part of our fight-or-flight system), our colours stick rigidly to their palette spot. But when epinephrine falls away, the brain loosens so that different circuits start to connect – prompting the emergence of memories, ideas and novel thoughts. Which is to say, that for our imaginations to bloom, we need to be completely free of circulating stress hormones.

"Nothing is quite as calming as the slow, contained flow of a canal"

So how do canals and towpaths fit in to Heilman's ideas of creativity? Well, a towpath requires no map-reading or navigation whatsoever. We simply step onto the path and follow it, walking for as long or as little as we need – many canal paths run for hundreds of miles, so we can amble until ideas drift into our calm, soothed minds – and safe in the knowledge that we can't possibly get lost, that we need do nothing but walk.

"This combination of water and slowness calms my mind"

It isn't just epinephrine that can impede imaginative thought. Studies have repeatedly found that the stress hormone cortisol can also suppress connections between remote brain regions.[4] Like epinephrine, cortisol rises (sometimes nine-fold) when we're stressed. According to neuroscientists, cortisol also disrupts navigation-related brain circuits, making an easy-to-follow route vital not only for those who want to think as creatively as possible but for those who are already stressed when they set off.[5] All of which comes to this: nothing is quite as calming as the slow, contained flow of a canal.

For Canal Poet Laureate Jo Bell, it's the slowness that matters. 'Everything is slow, from the water flow to the movement of barges,' she explained. 'This combination of water and slowness calms my mind, enabling me to apply the close scrutiny that poetry requires. Even cyclists and joggers are too hurried for a canal tow path.'[6]

"This blend of tranquil monotony and sporadic interest provides the perfect soil for germinating new ideas"

Creativity also requires solitude. As Heilman points out, 'Creative ideas are produced by looking "inside".' Anything that inhibits 'looking inside' threatens our ability to think imaginatively. This doesn't just mean that we need an easy-to-navigate landscape for our ideas to happily ferment. It also means we need to be alone. A chatty friend, impenetrable crowds, sudden noise – indeed too much distraction of any sort – take us out of ourselves, making it more difficult to hear our inner voice. Unsurprisingly, Heilman adds that negligible 'levels of arousal' are vital for spurring creative thoughts. Again, a canal ticks the box – offering long stretches of quiet, uniform track interspersed with (usually) predictable distraction, much of which repeats (the odd barge, bridge, sluice gate and lock, for example). This blend of tranquil monotony and sporadic interest provides the perfect soil for germinating new ideas – just enough activity to stop our brain becoming bored, but not quite enough to continually interrupt the meanderings of our mind.

Nor is this all. Psychologists think there's something about the linear aspect of a canal (as opposed to a twisting, meandering river, or an ebbing and flowing ocean) that appeals deeply to the human brain. We like straight lines because we can easily measure them, because they tell our brain that we are moving efficiently towards our destination, because we are not distracted or unsettled by what might be lurking around the corner. Despite the generally accepted human preference for looking at curves (see Chapter 4, 'Rolling

Hills'), we also carry a fondness for continuous straight lines. According to researchers at Penn State University, we like their simplicity, symmetry and orderliness.[7]

"Direction and certitude focus the creative mind"

So, as we walk a towpath – utterly relaxed because our phone is turned off and there's no need to make a single navigational decision, with our brain imaginatively loosened by dwindling stress hormones – we also feel the surety and purpose of a perfectly straight pair of lines taking us directly to an end point. Of course, not all towpaths are perfectly straight – the Oxford Canal route is notoriously winding – but many have a methodical linearity that, combined with their slow pace, is instinctively appreciated by the human brain. As canal walker and acclaimed poet Jonathan Davidson, told me, 'The canal feels as if it's giving me that little bit of direction and certitude, enough to focus the creative mind. Like a canal, a poem has to be made to go somewhere.'

Research into the effects of shapes and lines on the human brain is in its infancy, so rather than rely on the work of pioneering researchers (or even a single poet), why not experiment on yourself? I did exactly that, a few years ago when I spent ten days walking from Bordeaux to Toulouse, beside the River Garonne and the Canal de Garonne. I began by following the river, but found myself switching more and more frequently to the canal towpath. The (tidal) river meandered madly, which meant entire stretches of path had been washed away. I could not tell at what points the path would peter out, while some of the meanders meant miles of additional walking. At a point in my life when I longed for direction and stability, the call of the canal grew louder and louder.

Eventually I swapped the circuitous, empty river for the straight-lined canal with its houseboats and dog walkers. Here, ideas, images and phrases came to me, but in a way that seemed mysteriously ordered, even page-ready. As if the clean lines of the canal had shaped and structured my words. Although I lost my heart to the river, I lost my head to the canal, eventually arriving in Toulouse with a new sense of purpose and a notebook crammed with ideas, jottings, even a couple of poems.

And herein lies yet another benefit of a flat, even towpath: we can jot down – as we walk – all those brilliantly inventive ideas tumbling through our canal-calmed minds.

notes

Not sure where to start? Try the UK's Seven Wonders of the Waterways – a list created half a century ago featuring some of Britain's most impressive canals. For more information, visit canalrivertrust.org.uk, a fantastic resource for any canal walker.

The US is home to a number of iconic canal cities, including Cape Coral on Florida's Gulf Coast, Fort Lauderdale, Chesapeake City, Birmingham in Alabama, Portland in Oregon and San Antonio in Texas. For a longer route, try the historic, 400-mile-long Erie Canal through upstate New York.

Some of the most interesting canals are found in cities – from Venice to Amsterdam, Hamburg, Amiens, Berlin, Bruges and Paris. Birmingham, however, has more canal paths than any of its more famous peers.

Look out for canal museums, including Chesapeake City's C&D Canal Museum, London's Canal Museum and Amsterdam's Museum of the Canals.

The Canal du Midi in the South of France is one of the world's earliest and most impressive canals – and the most celebrated in France. Its towpaths are ideal for a long-distance, mapless hike, and perfect for anyone wanting to free their inner historian, engineer or poet.

Canals are often at their best in spring and autumn and at their busiest in August. Opt for August if you want plenty of hustle and bustle, and other months if you want peace and quiet.

Cortisol has a strong diurnal rhythm, typically peaking in the hour after we wake, then gradually tapering off over the course of a day.[8] To be fully free from its inhibiting grip, walk the towpath in the afternoon or (if it's light) in the evening.

Not sure how long to walk for? A new study suggests that even a five-minute walk results in more original ideas than being sedentary.[9] According to neuroscientist Dr Chong Chen, 'just a few minutes of walking . . . can enhance creative thinking'.[10]

Worried about being too alone? Canals can vary hugely from the absolutely deserted to those bustling with barges, cyclists and walkers. Find a busy urban canal with plenty of local activity, or walk in August. And never walk for ideas if you feel fearful or uncomfortable – fear triggers adrenaline and cortisol, halting all creativity in its tracks.

Most towpaths are suitable for wheelchairs, children's bikes and pushchairs, making them well-suited to those in need of inspiration but also needing to accommodate wheels.

No need for walking poles or hefty hiking boots on a towpath. A pair of trainers will do the job.

Most canals start and/or finish in towns and cities, meaning you won't need to ponder over petrol and parking or fret about adding to the burden of pollution. Take public transport to the start and consider making it a round trip by using one of the many bridges.

Take water and snacks – some towpaths are surprisingly devoid of places to shop, eat and drink.

Canals are invariably free of traffic, making them peaceful enough to hear your own genius ideas. Better yet, the lack of pollution may well build your creativity muscle. Worrying research from the University of Cambridge found that companies based in densely polluted areas came up with fewer innovations, concluding that 'pollution makes societies less creative'.[11]

For minimal distraction, put your phone away. Instead, take a tiny notebook and pencil to jot down whatever words come to you, poetic or otherwise. Prepare to be surprised!

The even terrain of a towpath makes it ideal for a faster pace, but (if it's ideas you're after) resist the temptation to move too fast. When we push our bodies to excess, we flood ourselves with imagination-killing stress hormones.

CANAL TOWPATHS

While canal towpaths are particularly suited to sparking new ideas, the lack of required navigation and map-reading (and the lack of hill-ish exertion) makes them perfect for any walk where the aim is to reflect, think and ponder.

Walking beside moving water – be it canal or stream – can help relieve feelings of loneliness as well as boosting our supplies of the happiness hormone, serotonin (see Chapter 10, 'Lakes').

The biodiversity of canals, combined with their architectural interest (from barges to bridges and aqueducts), make towpaths perfect for kindling the curiosity of older children.

Canal towpaths are – in my experience – also the very best routes for becoming immersed in a podcast or audiobook.

Ecotones

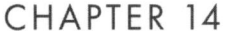

The Mind-Boggling
Brilliance of Birds

'The robins are singing sweetly. Now for my walk . . .'

DOROTHY WORDSWORTH, *JOURNALS OF DOROTHY WORDSWORTH*, VOL. 1, MARCH 1802

- - - - - - - -

DEFINITION: A region of transition between two biological communities or habitats, often richer in species than either.

BENEFITS FOR: Anxiety. Confusion. Those in need of mental stimulation. Those in need of certainty and predictability.

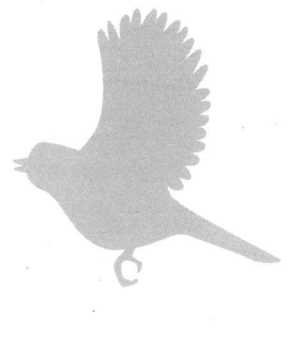

CHAPTER 14

I n January 2019, two men appeared on BBC's *Winterwatch* where, to the surprise of viewers, they candidly shared details of earlier attempts to take their own lives. One – the well-known TV presenter Chris Packham – explained that his dogs had saved his sanity and his life. The other – a writer called Joe Harkness – described how birds had been his saviour.

'I was talked down from the loft hatch where I thought my life would end,' he explains. 'Later, therapy and medication helped ... but nothing came close to my experiences with birds.' Joe's first epiphany struck as he was out walking. He looked up and saw two buzzards 'regally displaying above a tree line. They were so majestic. Watching them swoop, rise and dive was mesmerising. And oh, how I wanted to fly with them and be liberated from the shackles of my mind.'

As Joe gave up alcohol and began putting his life back together, he started noticing the birds around him. 'Birds are like an anchor to the present moment, a form of mindfulness,' he says. 'They gave me a sense of connection, to nature, to other birders, but most importantly to my inner self.'

Birdwatching isn't sedentary, adds Joe, who documented his return to health in his bestselling book, *Bird Therapy*. 'We move between habitats and locations, carrying optics and cameras. Sometimes I can walk for miles.'

We know that domestic animals and pets reduce stress,

loneliness and anxiety.[1] But, although much less studied, wild animals appear to do exactly the same. In 2009, researchers observed and interviewed nearly 4,000 passers-by interacting with wildlife in a series of US urban parks. Their subsequent analysis showed that, for 90 per cent of people, wildlife encounters enhanced their walk.[2]

"Encounters with wildlife enable us to step outside of ourselves"

A decade later, two researchers interviewed several hundred people on the subject of their recent encounters with marine wildlife. As they collated the findings, they were struck by the repeated use of words like 'eye-opening', 'humbling', 'magical' and 'magnificent'. Interviewees spoke of profound feelings of 'connection' and many talked of being 'changed' by their encounter. But the greatest epiphanies took place when participants sensed that an animal had acknowledged or witnessed them.[3]

Somehow, encounters with wildlife enable us to step outside

of ourselves. We cease to see a world that revolves around us, seeing instead a world in which we are simply part of a vast pulsing web of life. As the researchers involved in this experiment explained, 'Feelings of love, belonging, fulfilment and perspective were linked with the human–animal experience.'[4]

"Observing life in the wild alters not only our mood but our biology"

Over and over again, evidence suggests that when we interact with wildlife, we exist more fully, we live more richly. This extraordinary sense of connection was eloquently expressed by writer Helen Macdonald, who described these moments as those 'in which the world stutters, turns and fills with unexpected meaning'.[5]

But we don't respond solely with our emotions. We also respond with our bodies. In the last couple of years, researchers have started using technology – from blood and saliva tests to EEG and fMRI – to study the physiological impact of watching non-human life. Again, the results have been remarkable. Even watching fish swimming has been found to lower blood pressure and heart rate.[6] Observing life in the wild alters not only our mood but our biology.

Significantly, these feelings aren't fleeting – they endure. When researchers analysed data from 1,300 people who had uploaded thousands of diary entries in which they reflected on their environment and their wellbeing, birds were the single most significant source of joy.[7] On hearing or seeing a bird, participants felt a jolt of joy which persisted for hours after the bird encounter. Ryan Hammond at the Institute of Psychiatry, Psychology and Neuroscience at King's College London refers to this as a 'time-lasting link'. To boot, birds brought as much joy to the already contented as to those diagnosed with depression.

Similar results were found when a team of German researchers investigated the practice of birdwatching among residents in sixty-five nursing homes. Here the research team had two specific questions: firstly, could watching birds really make residents happier and healthier? And secondly, could it lead to sustainable and lasting changes to a resident's mental and physical health?

Again, the answer to both questions was a resounding yes. After eight weeks of birdwatching, the residents – many of whom were frail, unwell or in the throes of dementia – were moving more, their memory skills had improved, and they were interacting with each other more frequently. 'We found that cognitive resources, mobility, and biopsychosocial health improved,' explained the lead researcher, 'even among residents with severe cognitive and physical deficiencies.' The researchers also found that, instead of growing bored, the more that residents birdwatched, the more attached to the practice they became,[8] creating a sort of virtuous circle of wellbeing.

"Listening to birdsong reduced stress"

Nor do we need to see wildlife to feel happier. Even six-minute audio clips of birdsong reduced feelings of anxiety, depression and paranoia. 'Listening to birdsong through headphones hit the same pathways beneficial for mental wellbeing,' Hammond told the *Washington Post*, confirming that birdsong reduced stress by lowering blood pressure and cortisol levels. Meanwhile, listening to traffic made people feel more depressed.[9]

"The more diverse and varied the birdsong, the happier we become"

Nor is it just birds that lift our spirits. New evidence suggests that observing butterflies can be as soothing and hopeful as birdwatching. When a team of researchers surveyed people involved in an annual butterfly count, they noted that participants had lower levels of anxiety and an enhanced sense of 'nature connectedness' during and afterwards. In fact, anxiety levels fell by 10 per cent, even after a mere fifteen minutes of butterfly observation.[10]

Perhaps most pertinently of all, the latest research indicates that the more diverse and varied the birdsong (and wildlife in general), the happier we become. This is hardly surprising, given the brain's love of novelty (see Chapter 16, 'Outlands'). But what really took researchers' breath away was just how much we value diverse and varied wildlife. When German researchers sought to put a price on the biodiversity of birdlife, they concluded 'that the effect of bird species richness on life-satisfaction may be of similar magnitude to that of income'.[11] People, it appeared, were prepared to sacrifice money rather than live with fewer breeds of bird.

So where should we walk to 'meet' wildlife, to have the sorts of life-enriching bird encounters that saved Joe Harkness? According to Emma Robertshaw of the Wildlife Trusts, 'Healthy wetlands, healthy peatlands and Atlantic rainforests are probably the most biodiverse habitats (in the UK). But species-rich meadows can be amazing too. Even better, head for the scrubby woodland-grassland edge of a marsh and take in birds of prey, waders, reed-dwelling birds, deer, hare, and you might be lucky enough to have an otter or weasel cross your path too.'

Scientists have a name for edge areas like these, spaces where ecosystems overlap or morph into one another: ecotones. Or edgelands.* Various studies have shown that species richness tends to peak in ecotonal areas. In fact, these biodiversity hotspots, the fringes that lie between two landscapes, can even trigger the evolution of new species. When biologists began studying the wildlife roaming the wooded fringe where the rainforests of Cameroon meet savannah, they discovered that little greenbuls (small, green birds) living on the forest edge

---

* The term 'edgelands' is commonly used to describe the strips of land where suburban factories and housing estates spill over into semi-rural scrubland, but here I use the term as a synonym for an ecotone.

sang at a pitch unlike that of their jungle counterparts, despite being the same species. The birds had altered their pitch to overcome the ambient noise peculiar to the forest edge. They had also evolved to have heavier bodies, longer legs, lengthier wings and deeper bills, which the biologists hypothesised were necessary traits in the more open and exposed environment of the forest fringe.[12]

We're unlikely to spot any newly evolved birds in our own ecotones, but look and listen out for particular birds: studies show that some varieties are more pleasing to our eye and ear than others. We typically like smaller, non-aggressive birds, and we're very partial to colourful birds. Joe Harkness realised that he too was partial to diversity of birdlife and habitat as well as to colour. In fact, when he moved to a new birding location, Joe knew instinctively that the place wasn't right: 'It didn't inspire me ... it often left me feeling confused and anxious.' For weeks Joe couldn't understand why his new spot – a wetland site with a history of wildlife monitoring – didn't beckon to him as his old 'patch' had. And then he put his finger on it: the new location didn't have the same variety of habitats, and that meant fewer birds. 'I realised that a restorative environment ... requires a convergence of habitats and microenvironments,' he writes in *Bird Therapy*. For him that meant an ecotone of myriad habitats: 'heathland, wildflower meadow, valley mire, mixed woodland and masses of dense scrub'.

Later, Joe identified another reason for the profound influence birdlife had on his state of mind. 'The logic and consistency of birds made sense,' he explains. 'They appeared at predictable times in predictable places. Their comings and goings were repetitive and comforting. They gave a rhythm to my life, easing my anxiety.'

Just as Joe was publishing *Bird Therapy*, Professor Miles Richards was investigating 'joy-rating' as a means of identifying the birds that bring most joy. Richards found that 'the smaller and more colourful the bird, the more joy it brought'. His research identified tits, robins and goldfinches as the greatest 'joy-bringers', while crows, magpies and pigeons languished at the bottom of the bird popularity table.

But infinitely more important than this was Richards' discovery that 'joy-rating' made birdwatching more calming and restorative than simply observing, counting and logging. After thirty minutes of watching birds and engaging with how the bird made them feel, respondents reported dramatically falling anxiety.

How so? Richards thinks that 'activating a sense of joy heightens the benefits birdwatching brings', leading to feelings of calm (slower, steadier breathing and heart rate, for example) that blunt anxiety. When we 'notice and rate feelings of joy', says Richards, we become happier. Moreover, just thirty minutes of watching and joy-rating led 'to a direct and measurable improvement in wellbeing'. It also led to a much higher feeling of connection to nature, compared with a baseline group who merely recorded facts and figures.

"Birdsong improves mood, mental awareness and the ability to concentrate"

I have one final theory for why certain birds calm and enchant us. The sound of birdsong is the sound of safety. A sort of primal safety cue. Birds only sing and chatter when they feel safe enough to declare their presence and share their location. Squirrels know this, as Ohio ornithologists discovered after exposing grey squirrels to the sound of a predator immediately followed by the sound of birdsong. Squirrels that heard bird chatter following a hawk's call returned to normal levels of watchfulness more quickly than squirrels exposed to silence after a hawk's call. The casual chatter of birds, said the ornithologists, appeared to indicate safety for the squirrels.[13] I think we humans recognise this too: landscapes bereft of bird chatter can feel ominously unsettling.

And perhaps this explains why researchers have also found that some birdsong improves mood, mental awareness and the ability to concentrate.[14]

notes

Ecotones are everywhere – river banks, dunes, where the rim of a forest meets surrounding fields, where fresh water merges with salt water and, yes, where urban sprawl meets rural wasteland. Seek them out, keep quiet, move slowly. Ideally, take binoculars and/or a pop-up hide.

The decline in bird species diversity and abundance may be affecting our collective mental health in ways we haven't fully untangled. Lobby to protect our birds. Feed them where appropriate. Cherish them.

In the last few years 53 per cent of our native plants – all too often the source of food for birds – have declined, suggesting that they too need our protection. Avoid pesticides and lights in your garden and create wilderness corners where insects can thrive.

Not all birds are equal. We humans are not quite as fond of crows, pigeons and seagulls, for example. Don't expect these birds to have the same mood-lifting effects as songbirds.

Songbirds typically like scrubland, brambles and hedgerows. Use a birdsong app to identify them (I like the Merlin app), and tune into how they make you feel.

No birds? Listen to birdsong online – even this can lift mood and dampen feelings of depression.

Meanwhile, continue lobbying for the protection of wild areas. Studies make it quite clear that we are happier in places where we can hear 'the sounds of wildlife, such as birdsong'.[15]

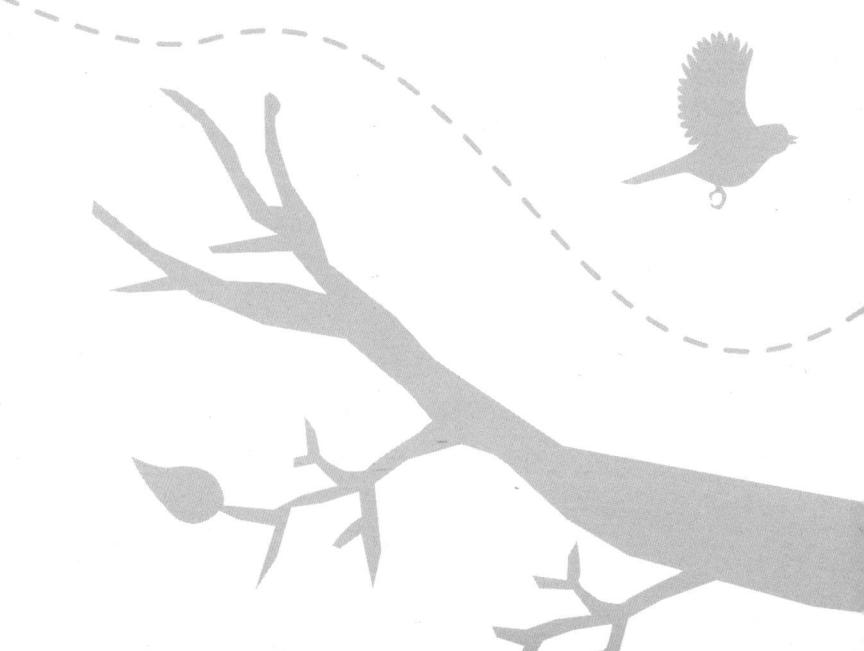

Urban Parks and Gardens

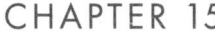

Communal, Clean, Curative

'A mile from Bonn is a garden . . . planted with thick and lofty groves . . . On some days half the inhabitants of Bonn are to be seen in this garden, mingling in the promenade.'

ANN RADCLIFFE, *A JOURNEY MADE IN THE SUMMER OF 1794*

DEFINITION: An urban area that offers respite, rest, recreation, education, exercise, inspiration or enjoyment to residents of, and visitors to, that urban area.

BENEFITS FOR: Sickness, convalescence and recovery; loneliness; frailty; urban overload and nature deficiency.

Twenty years ago, my husband lay close to death in a London hospital. After a week in a coma, he was moved out of intensive care and into a succession of wards. Double pneumonia followed by adrenal-gland failure had left him too weak to walk – or so we thought. The hospital staff were keen for him to stay in bed, but he was young and, as he grew stronger, he insisted on getting out of bed and walking with me up and down the corridors. From the corridors we progressed to the small smoking zone at the front of the hospital. Here, we ambled up and down as smokers puffed beside us and juggernauts lumbered past. Eventually we found a small park and he walked there – the only hospital patient to be hobbling slowly up and down the rose garden.

Last year a team of Spanish researchers decided to investigate the wisdom of hospital bed rest. What would happen, they asked, if hospital patients spent less time in bed and a little more time moving. More importantly, to see the best possible results, how much time would patients need to spend moving and what sort of movement should they do? The researchers began combing methodically through all the studies and papers published during the previous two decades. From the 4,000 inpatients surveyed – all admitted for serious illness – they gleaned that not only was movement vital to a good recovery, but that the most appropriate form of movement was walking.

Walking was more than 80 per cent effective, they concluded, with an optimal duration of around seventy minutes a day, and a minimal duration of twenty-five minutes a day. Inpatients that ambled daily, they added, could avoid 'post-hospital syndrome', an umbrella term for the vulnerability and frailty that often strike after patients are discharged. Too much bed rest, they noted, often resulted in a greater chance of patients subsequently being readmitted, needing nursing-home care, falling ill again, or simply dying.

For the first time, the age-old concept of complete bed rest had been turned on its head. As I read over this report, I thought back to my husband's hospital corridor potters, the lack of a hospital garden and the subsequent lifeline offered by our London parks. He didn't return to work for another three months, but during that time our local park became an indispensable place of safety and calm where he could see other people, play with our toddlers, drink from the fountain and rest on a bench when needed.

Parks and public gardens are the vital lungs of our cities – and not just for hospital escapees. A surge of recent studies has made it plain just how invaluable the plain old (green) park is for every aspect of a city dweller's wellbeing.

CHAPTER 15

"Parks are vital spaces of sanctuary and connection, places in which to move, breathe, think, recover"

In 2021 researchers from the University of the West of England found that stress and anxiety levels among young people were reduced by between 14 per cent and 19 per cent after a fifteen-minute walk in an urban park, when compared with a street walk.[1] A study of men found that, after walking in a city park, their heart rate lowered, they felt calmer, more relaxed and less anxious.[2] A study of older walkers found 'significant decreases' in blood and pulse pressure while park walking, compared to pavement walking, which was deemed to have 'adverse effects on cardiovascular health'. And a Japanese study found a dramatic fall in 'tension-anxiety, anger, depression, fatigue and confusion', alongside increased feelings of vigour, among adults after walking Tokyo parks and gardens.[3]

Indeed, studies like this are now ten a penny: parks and public gardens are quite probably the most valuable asset of any urban area. As climate change threatens ever greater heat and discomfort, and as more and more of us live in flats, our parks will become vital spaces of sanctuary and connection, places in which to move, breathe, think, recover.

> "We typically walk further and for longer in *larger* parks with less hard surfacing and more greenery"

And yet not all parks are equal. A growing body of evidence makes it clear that some parks are more conducive to our happiness, health and serenity than others. In 2020, when researchers monitored people walking through different parks, they found that the park design 'had an immediate effect . . . different landscape types led to different physiological responses and mood states'. [4] How a park is designed, planted, constructed and cared for shapes our response, lifting or felling our mood within seconds.

So what sort of park should we look for? Like my recovering husband, most of us will make a beeline for our closest park. For those of us with more scope to travel, however, it's worth exploring further afield. And for those of us with local parks that haven't been generously invested in, let this chapter be the nudge we need to demand more from our city planners.

Size matters – we typically walk further and for longer in *larger* parks. We also walk further and for longer in parks with less hard surfacing and more greenery. For winter walks, that means a park with plenty of evergreen trees and foliage. Either way, your chosen park should have more foliage and less concrete. And while an abundance of greenery is consistently associated with instantly tumbling stress levels, we don't like it shoved into straggly clumps in corners, and we don't like it to look too unkempt. For women (many of whom, sadly, feel less safe than men in their local parks), greenery should enhance rather than obscure lines of sight.

When it comes to our emotional restoration, we like our parks to include water (fountains, ponds and lakes – and the larger the better, see Chapter 10 for why larger bodies of water make us happy). Studies show that we usually slow our pace when we encounter water in parks, suggesting that we appreciate spending time in its presence. Water also lures eyecatching wildlife, and we like some of that in our parks too – ducks, butterflies, birds (see Chapter 14, 'Ecotones' for why wildlife raises our spirits).

Water and wildlife aren't the only things that please us. Man-made structures (bridges, pergolas, gates) are also an important element in a restorative park, providing interest for our fizzing brains and fuel for our sense of curiosity. And perhaps also reminding us that parks – unlike genuine wilderness – are places inhabited by people.[5]

Above all, we like our parks and gardens to include mature woodland and flowers. Huge old trees and swathes of beautiful blooms are better for our emotional equilibrium than anything else – including cafés, benches, bridges and ponds (although these are vital too). According to studies in which walkers had their brains scanned while outdoors, deeper states of relaxation were reached in the presence of old trees when compared to young trees. Ancient trees calm and steady us. Perhaps it's because they release many more stress-countering phytoncides than their younger counterparts. Perhaps it's because their heft and girth speak to us of stability, constancy and certainty. Or perhaps their stature and majesty merely distract us from ourselves (see Chapter 1, 'Forests and Woodland').[6]

"We must find parks away from polluted air"

We like our urban parks well away from sources of noise pollution. When researchers investigated the popularity of parks in Beijing, they discovered very different responses according to the park's location. Those between huge ring roads elicited the least positive emotions.[7] For a park to provide the peace it promises, it must be free of traffic noise. Squealing brakes, sirens and car horns destroy any illusion of tranquillity.

A quiet park invariably means cleaner air – and we like to breathe fully in our parks. Not only does air pollution contribute to respiratory infections, heart disease, stroke and lung cancer, but a worrying number of studies now indicate that air pollution also affects brain chemistry, with many reporting a link between air pollution and illnesses of the mind – from dementia to depression and suicide. Some neurologists suspect that air pollution kick-starts a neuroinflammatory process in the brain. So, while we cannot always choose where we live or work, we must find parks away from polluted air.

Flowers also affect the emotions of most park visitors. We like their colour, their fractal shapes, the butterflies that feed from them. Flowers lift our spirits. They tug our feelings outwards. Unfortunately, too many parks plant the same blooms, although studies indicate that we like 'a diversity of flowers'.[8] We like their scent too. In fact, for many of us, the olfactory experience of a park can be as meaningful as what we see (see Chapter 6, 'Flowers and Meadows' for more on the astonishing effects of smell on our mood). Researchers investigating the most restorative places in a Mexican city found 'green' smellscapes to be as meaningful as 'visual contact with nature'.[9]

"Parks are arguably the single most important place in a city"

Finally, we're not particularly keen on large stretches of grass (although these are excellent places for sport, of course). One team of researchers found that the blood pressure and pulse rate of park walkers fell when near water but rose as soon as playing fields came into view. Unless you're kicking a ball, always choose a park over a playing field. And if your park is all grass and little more, lobby your local council for paths, plants, trees, water and a bench.

So what does all this mean? As a daily city-park walker of three decades, this reminds me to cherish my local park. But it also reminds me that city officials should be repeatedly nudged into improving our urban spaces. If your park is looking tired, uncared for, or has few restorative features, ask for some investment. Remind those in power that these are *our* spaces, the beating hearts of our communities. Arguably the single most important place in a city.

notes

We like our parks clean – pick up litter or lobby for bins if there are none.

It's imperative that parks feel safe – for everyone. If your park feels unsafe in any way, try to understand why (too many bushes? Too dark? Intimidating dogs? Poorly maintained benches?), then lobby for change.

Some urban parks are run by committees which can be joined by residents or non-officials. If you want to see change, get involved.

No park? Form a guerilla gardening group and plant up dead spaces and wastelands with seeds and weeds.

The pollution that seems to have greatest impact on our wellbeing – contributing not only to serious mental illness but to aggression, loss of emotional control and an inability to cope with crises – is thought to be particulate matter 2.5 (PM2.5), caused by traffic, factories and coal-fired power plants. Avoid parks in these areas and lobby your government for cleaner air (note: cities in Asia, Africa and the Middle East have by far the most polluted air).

Parks are a city's hardest-working space, catering for the different needs of thousands of people. Instead of berating the concrete corner reserved for skateboarders (for example), revel in the pulsing throb of humanity that makes its way here on a sunny Saturday afternoon. This is city life at its most joyous.

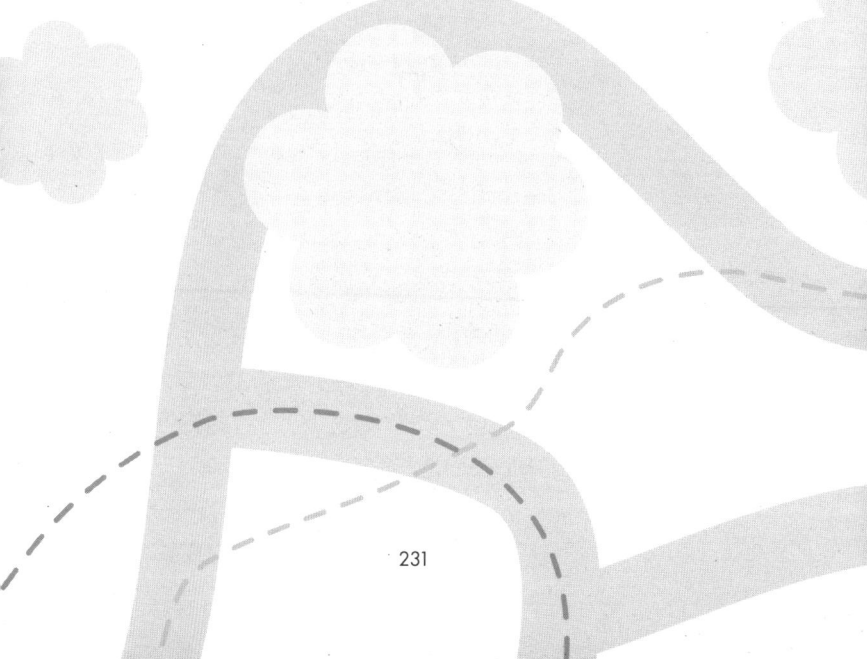

Outlands

In Search of
Sustainable Surprise

> 'He who cannot find wonder, mystery, awe, the sense of a new world and an undiscovered realm in the places by the Gray's Inn Road will never find those secrets elsewhere.'

ARTHUR MACHEN, *FAR OFF THINGS*

DEFINITION: The outlying districts or remote regions of a country. Formerly the outlying land of a feudal estate, usually granted to tenants. From Old English *ūtland*, meaning 'foreign country'.

BENEFITS FOR: Climate anxiety, restlessness, boredom, flight guilt, the urgent need for a change of scene, the time-poor and cash-strapped who long for the far-flung and exotic.

I n 2023 climate protester Deanna Coco had her fifteen-month jail sentence – for blocking a lane on Sydney Harbour Bridge – quashed by a judge who noted her 'diagnosed climate anxiety'. Sometimes called eco-anxiety or eco-anger, the stress brought on by climate change is very real. Researcher Susan Clayton has carried out several studies into climate anxiety and found it disproportionately high among young people, and particularly among young females. When she and her team surveyed 10,000 people aged sixteen to twenty-five across ten countries, 84 per cent claimed to be worried, with 59 per cent saying they were extremely worried. Almost half said their feelings about climate change negatively affected their daily life.[1]

Manifesting as 'depression, anxiety, and extreme emotions like sadness, anger, and fear',[2] 'eco-emotions are both visceral and numinous', researchers have noted.[3] Meanwhile climate anxiety often carries an insidious undertow of guilt. Indeed, over 50 per cent of those surveyed by Clayton's team reported feelings of eco-guilt.

Top of the list of guilt-inducing activities, for many of us, is travelling by aeroplane. In Sweden, flight shame now has its own word: *flygskam*. And yet, in the recent past, travelling to distant countries has often been a rite of passage – an opportunity to experience landscapes, weather conditions and cultures radically different from our own, to become jolted out of complacency, to encounter the new and the unknown, to escape the dull and quotidian.

"Our brains *need* – and often crave – novelty"

In truth, most of us relish novelty. When we encounter it, our brains reward us with a shot of dopamine, which is why it can feel so good, and why walkers who sought out new locations during the confines of Covid-19 often reported better mental health than those who stuck to the same old trail. Evolutionary biologists hypothesise that, as foraging hunters and nomads, we evolved to explore new terrain and were rewarded for doing so. The dopamine shot encouraged us to explore, without which Homo sapiens may never have survived.

"We are designed to explore"

So perhaps it's no surprise that our brains *need* – and often crave – novelty. Exposure to new things encourages the growth of new neurons, making travel a brain-expanding imperative. Our brains are particularly partial to spatial novelty, which has been shown to improve memory and learning. Studies have found that participants exposed to new places immediately before or after learning had better recall and understanding than participants who remained at their desks.[4] Meanwhile, older people who repeatedly encountered the new and novel lived for longer, while rat pups exposed to novel environments in the first three weeks of life were better able to learn for at least another year after exposure. As the authors of one study explained, 'Exploring new opportunities, seeking out new situations and exploring novel environments is a core trait of adaptive mammalian behavior.'[5] In other words, we are designed to explore.

"The unexpected can be found closer to home than we think"

You can probably see where I'm going here . . . for the last few decades, travel by plane – often to distant and very different locations – has provided much-needed change and excitement, frequently at ludicrously low prices, thanks to the emergence of budget airlines. Without the availability of cheap flights, few of us have either the time or the money to get anywhere far-flung or exotic. But when we forego flying, are we really giving up the opportunity of experiencing landscapes that are excitingly new and unfamiliar?

Not so fast. Studies have shown that it is mostly the *unexpectedness* of novelty that excites our minds. Fortunately, the unexpected can be found closer to home than we typically think. We don't necessarily need a long-haul, guilt-inducing flight to be jolted out of our mundane lives. As the writer Nick Hunt discovered.

Hunt had always loved the novelty and surprise of travel. Indeed, he loved it so much that he became a travel writer. But somewhere around 2018 he began feeling a growing sense of disquiet at 'the damage that travel can do'. Climate breakdown no longer felt like a distant future emergency but more like an imminent catastrophe. The 'chemical violence done to the stratosphere by flying' sickened him, while the disappearance of the landscapes of his childhood alarmed and distressed him. Instead, he began looking for 'transformative journeys' and 'transporting' landscapes that were closer to home.[6]

Hunt found many such landscapes were a mere bus ride away, ranging from Europe's largest expanse of shingle, to a Devon woodland that was more like a rainforest and felt like 'stepping into a primordial other-world', to a patch of Arctic tundra he described as 'out of place . . . an exclave of the Arctic stranded in Scotland'.

But it was the plain old shingle of Kent that first showed Hunt how very *local* the outlandish could be. 'Why go to the Sahara when you can visit Kent?' he wrote in *Outlandish: Walking Europe's Unlikely Landscapes*. On this vast expanse of Kentish pebbles, beneath the apocalyptic shadow of a nuclear power station, Hunt noted that 'the sky was not the English sky . . . With crimson light pouring over a scene of wind-whipped marram grass and the skeletons of boats, I experienced a moment of dislocation; suddenly I was not in England but in a North American wasteland . . . it was briefly enough to jolt me free of time and space. I found myself transported.'

"Outlands can shock us out of today and into 'deep time'"

Later, Hunt travelled by train to walk other outlands – a jungle in Poland, a desert in Spain, steppes in Hungary, fjords in Ireland, and 'badlands' in France and Italy known locally as the *calanques* and the *calanchi*. But he maintains that outlands of sorts – 'geological oddities . . . portals to elsewhere' – can be found in the least likely and most local of places. Moreover, these geographical anomalies did more than jolt Hunt into new spaces, they often jolted him through time, enabling him to glimpse both the distant past and a possible future. 'Thousands of years stretched between the [Dungeness] flints whose striking once sparked fire and the nuclear power station whose waste will last for centuries more . . . for a moment we stood between the past and the future,' he wrote. Outlands can shock us, he suggests, out of today and into 'deep time'.

As I researched this chapter, my daughter and I walked 22 km from Rye in East Sussex to Dungeness on the outermost corner of Kent. Within a few hours we were among some of the most bizarre and rare of British plants and lichens, heaving our booted feet over miles and miles of shingle with the empty power station looming eerily overhead and gunfire from a nearby military base exploding in the distance. The place felt oddly surreal in a way we hadn't expected. Nudged from our everyday worlds, we pondered nuclear power, the bleached grey lichens that sprung directly from rocks, the troughs of ocean-sculpted shells and bones that neatly lined the shingle, the windswept wooden cabins inhabited by artists, who displayed their driftwood sculptures from their bleak, stony gardens.

> "Walking a local outland
> is an inexpensive,
> time-saving cure for
> restiveness"

Hunt was right: this place felt less like a daily walk than 'a pilgrimage into the imagination'. We returned exhilarated, exhausted and very slightly smug. After all, we had (ad)ventured into a startlingly exotic landscape without a whiff of air travel, our carbon footprint intact. Any Londoner could have done exactly the same, courtesy of a train and a bus. My daughter and I talked about our Dungeness walk for weeks to come. It seemed to have settled into our memories as brightly and sharply as neuroscientists had promised. More significantly, it showed us that we could be moved, rejuvenated and 'jolted' without the need to board a plane.

Of course you don't need to be suffering from acute climate anxiety to venture into outlandish landscapes. Walking a local outland is also an inexpensive, time-saving cure for restiveness – those days, weeks and months when, for whatever reason, you crave weirdness, surprise, adventure, the unexpected. When your pockets aren't deep enough, your annual holiday not long enough to go to the Arctic, the desert, the rainforest or the grand canyons and fjords of *elsewhere*.

But why are outlandish places so memorably jolting, so imaginatively exciting? Part of the answer might lie in how our brains respond to the surprise and shock inherent in discovering, for example, a desert wasteland among the orchards of Kent. When researchers at the Massachusetts Institute of Technology studied the brains of mice startled by sudden and unexpected change, they noticed that a region called the locus coeruleus produced an immediate gush of noradrenaline which subsequently changed the behaviour of many of the mice. Not only were these startled mice then more likely to take chances, but they were also infused with a new vigour. Tests showed that the noradrenaline had travelled to the brain's motor cortex, an area that sends out nerve impulses to stimulate muscle movement.

Other experiments revealed that the surprised mice learned new behaviours more quickly and improved their accuracy at set tasks, prompting the researchers to wonder if surprise-induced noradrenaline might play an important role in helping us learn from the unexpected. The element of surprise, concluded the researchers, served to 'momentarily increase goal-oriented attention'.[7] See the notes below for my thoughts on how this can benefit outland walkers.

notes

A novel environment is only novel and unexpected if we haven't yet experienced it: we can increase the unexpectedness of a walk and a landscape by *not* poring over online pictures and maps before we go. The less you've seen in advance, the better . . .

We often remember the unexpected with greater clarity. These places can magically whittle themselves into our memory with lasting effects. So put the iPhone/camera away and let the novelty (and your brain) do its extraordinary work.

Take a pencil and sketchbook with you: drawing, or describing the landscape in (handwritten) words, will store the experience more deeply in our memory.[8]

"Outlands can be found just about anywhere"

Other UK rainforests include Cwm Mynach in Snowdonia and Crinan Wood in Argyll, Scotland, where 245 species of lichen have recently been recorded. Sadly, these landscapes are now very fragile and in need of urgent protection.

My own personal outlands (all of which can be reached by train or ferry) include Bohemia's labyrinthine rock caves, Albania's pelican-populated Karavasta lagoon, and La Gomera's Garajonay National Park, which contains a vast and ancient laurel forest.

More prosaically and less literally, outlands can be found just about anywhere. Botanical gardens, disused quarries, gorges, canyons and rock formations, even forgotten cemeteries, are often home to astonishingly unfamiliar plants, fungi and insects, which can startle us out of our usual ways of seeing. And all the better if we chance upon them, when their sheer unexpectedness can yield the same catalysing effect, kindling our brain, lighting our imagination and making us feel the childlike thrill of an explorer.

Be prepared to explore, to take the byways rather than the highways. Sometimes it's when we're lost that we come across the least predictable places, spaces and encounters.

Less social hours can help a landscape suddenly seem more mysteriously other. Standing stones emerging from a lonely dawn mist or rippling with silver moonlight are more likely to jolt us from the everyday than the very same stones surrounded by sunshiney, selfie-wielding crowds.

Dramatic shifts in weather can also render a familiar landscape unfamiliar. Storms (and the ethereal light that often precedes them), snow and frost, for example, can transform a location. Take these opportunities to revisit a favourite place and let its newness invigorate and inspire you.

When we experience surprise and shock, a cascade of chemicals (cortisol, dopamine, and especially noradrenaline) rushes through our brain, making us more alert, vigilant, energised. These are excellent opportunities to take very close notice of the landscape. Our brains are primed to pay extra attention when we're surprised, and so we are more likely to notice – and remember – things that would normally pass us by.

These are also opportunities (should we need them) to pick up the pace. With extra dopamine, cortisol and adrenaline circulating in our systems, we should be able to walk further and faster.

There are lots of outdoor companies making ethical and eco-friendly clothing and hiking boots, often using recycled materials. Take a reusable water bottle, DEET-free insect repellent and ocean-friendly mineral sunscreen. And remember that, while walking, your carbon footprint is negligible.

Distance Routes and Pilgrim Paths

The Psychology of Flow

'I walk until given shelter, fast
until given food . . . I usually
average twenty-five miles a day.'

PEACE PILGRIM

DEFINITION: A long, rural/wildish track
designated for walkers, often long distance, meaning
the walk lasts multiple days. Trail lengths range from
a few miles to hundreds of miles and typically cover
multiple terrains/landscapes.

BENEFITS FOR: Emotional turmoil, confusion,
anxiety, a restless desire for change, a broken heart.

CHAPTER 17

When Lara Evans' best friend unexpectedly took his own life, Lara was at a loss. 'I was devastated,' she told me. 'I couldn't understand why, and I was tormented by my own failure to save him from himself. For weeks I ruminated, until one day I couldn't bear the endlessly churning recriminations any longer. I knew that I had to outwalk my own destructive thoughts. I decided to walk the Camino, even though I'd never walked for more than a few miles before and I'd never walked alone.'

Lara arrived at the start of the route both anxious and lighter in her mind. 'Just knowing that I was embarking on a pilgrimage made me feel better. I also felt as if I was honouring my friend's memory in a way that was worthy of him. I knew he would be my walking companion, but, yes, I was very nervous.'

When Lara returned a fortnight later, she had clocked up over 200 miles. More importantly, she had shed much of her confusion and guilt along the way. 'There was something about walking day after day . . . a simplicity, a rhythm, a paring-back of life to its bare essentials. With everything stripped back to the contents of my rucksack, and with a constant sense of forward momentum, the distress that had hounded me for so long seemed to melt into a more manageable sadness.'

"The longer the walk, the more marked were the effects on 'mental distress'"

Lara is one of millions who, each year, undertakes a pilgrimage or a long-distance hike at a time of extreme emotional pain. For millennia, we humans have embarked on very long walks in an attempt to answer some of the most profound questions of life. And for many of us, only a very long walk – day after day – can provide the time, space and solitude necessary to untangle the bleakest of experiences. But why is an extended route so effective at helping us cope with emotional distress? And why should we choose our route with care?

"Long distance walks enable us to enter a liminal, or transformational, space"

In 2021 a team of Danish psychologists decided to investigate the alleged psychotherapeutic properties of long walks. They wanted to know if a very long walk really shifted mood and mindset. After reviewing all the studies of distance walking, the results were clear: very long walks were 'a remedy against mental health issues', ameliorating stress, depression and anxiety. Qualitative data suggested that the longer the walk, the more marked were the effects on 'mental distress'.[1]

To test out these findings, they then interviewed (in great depth) a group of middle-aged adults who had recently returned from walking for several days. The researchers concluded that 'long-distance walks [enabled people] to enter a liminal, or transformational, space . . . helpful, or perhaps even therapeutic, in situations where personal transformation is required'.

"We walk into a mental state of openness"

Earlier studies had borne this out, with many walkers reporting dramatic life changes after hiking a lengthy route. But the Danish psychologists were still puzzled. Why, they pondered, might a long-distance walk help someone psychologically? They suspected that part of the answer might lie in the space accorded by a long walk during which we *stay* with our pain. A long-distance walk 'provides room; room to think, to remember, to feel what one is feeling, for as long as the feeling persists', they wrote, adding that simply putting one foot in front of the other makes us feel as if we are *doing* something, taking (a very simple and undemanding) action of sorts.

And yet what most struck the Danish psychologists was the distance walkers' state of mind, which they called 'mental openness'. This, they decided, 'was the crucial characteristic and defining feature' of a long-distance walk – a state of mind enabled by both the psychological distance of the destination and the lack of preoccupation with reaching it. Distance walkers, they wrote, were effectively 'walking into a mental state of openness', and this openness was fuel for the existential transformation that so many pilgrims or distance hikers subsequently experienced.

Mental openness also appears to act as an amplifier for flow, the powerfully altered state of consciousness identified by psychologist Mihaly Csikszentmihalyi in the 1970s. Csikszentmihalyi described flow as an optimal state of consciousness where we feel and perform at our best.[2] During flow, we are so utterly engrossed in what we're doing that we lose track of time, of the world around us. Researchers describe it as a highly rewarding, almost euphoric psychological state. Flow 'guru' Steven Kotler describes it quite simply as 'the time when we feel most alive'.[3]

Although flow has been discussed for over fifty years, scientists are only now beginning to unpick the precise alterations in brain activity that enable and sustain it. According to dozens of tests using EEG, MEG* and fMRI, the brain in flow has a very particular neurobiology, in which some brain parts are activated while others go into partial hibernation. Researchers speculate that the brain in flow is subject to altered neural oscillations, changed routes of connectivity, and the activations (and deactivations) of specific brain regions, alongside rising and falling neurochemicals. Indeed, several neuroscientists have found the 'flowing brain' to be remarkably similar to the deeply meditating brain or the brain on psychedelic drugs.[4]

During flow states, levels of neurochemicals like dopamine and noradrenaline are heightened. Researchers think feel-fantastic endocannabinoids (see Introduction) may 'be something of a master neuromodulator' when it comes to the flow state.[5] In fact, mounting evidence suggests that our

---

* Magnetoencephalography, which records magnetic activity in the brain.

endocannabinoid system plays a significant role in the onset of flow. And when our endocannabinoids are in full swing, the brain part sometimes called our fear or threat-detection hub (the amygdala) is shunted into semi-hibernation. Think of those circulating endocannabinoids as harmonious classical music drowning out the endless wail of passing sirens (our amygdala).

"Distance walking often kindles a state of flow"

Distance walking often kindles a state of flow: as far back as 2005, researchers reported that over 60 per cent of the Appalachian Trail walkers they interviewed had experienced flow, adding that 'for the majority of them it was a daily occurrence'.[6] The continuous experience of flow may explain why so many studies have linked long-distance walking to improved mental health.[7] In fact, Kotler thinks that walking in nature is an ideal means of entering flow, because it deactivates the prefrontal cortex (the brain region that likes to analyse, organise, regulate and plan). Turning down the volume of this brain part is a necessary step in achieving flow, he says.

The latest studies suggest that a number of specific factors can precipitate the onset of flow, including: novelty, complexity, unpredictability and a sense of challenge; clear goals or sense of purpose; an element of risk; some form of embodiment or sensual immersion.

More interesting still, researchers suspect that flow requires an early injection of stress. For Lara, this was supplied by her anxiety at the prospect of walking alone in an unknown country.[8] Indeed, distance walking meets many of the flow-inducing criteria listed above, from its element of challenge and unpredictability (the weather, for example) to its physicality and strong sense of directional purpose. Kotler adds risk and novelty to his daily walk by 'weaving between trees or running fast downhill'. But on an unfamiliar distance trail, every corner carries an element of flow-inducing risk and uncertainty.

Recently it's become apparent that the experience of flow yields long-lasting effects. Even after returning to our more usual state of mind, flow leaves its fingerprints: we feel happier, our life has a greater sense of meaning, we're more motivated, more empathetic, more resilient. Think of it as personal post-flow growth. Guy Hayward, co-founder of the British Pilgrimage Trust, credits the *duration* of a pilgrimage: 'Each additional day adds to the repeated circadian rhythm so that old emotions start to bubble up and heal,' he says. 'Loose emotional ends are tied up, meaning we return changed in some way. The physical act of walking is literal bodily flow through space and time, which helps our mental flow.'[9]

Meanwhile, short-term effects include an increase in creativity and insight. In fact, Kotler has found that creativity while in flow increases by 400 per cent.

"Regular changes of scenery can help us find resolution"

So why do location and landscape matter when it comes to finding flow as we distance walk? Flow-like states come most readily, apparently, when walkers are alone in challenging, scenic or meaningful locations. The less familiar these locations are, the more challenging they will be. And yet if the terrain is too challenging, fear and anxiety will override flow. The chance to meet others will temper fear, so well-marked routes where other hikers are passing or where villages and houses are skirted can aid rather than hinder the flow state.

To maintain a sense of novelty and unpredictability, constantly changing scenery is a prerequisite. Indeed, some psychologists think that regular changes of scenery (a route that covers multiple landscapes, for example) can help us find resolution. 'Through new perspectives, walkers may find new solutions or new meaning,' explained Dr Rob Saunders in his study of personal transformation through long-distance walking.[10]

Of course, most long-distance routes inevitably pass through multiple landscapes, while most traditional pilgrimage routes bisect villages and places of worship where pilgrims historically stayed overnight. Distancing oneself from familiar landscapes can provide the opportunity to reflect from a different perspective. 'The further away I get, the more I see,' wrote Sarah Marquis in her memoir of distance walking, *Wild by Nature*.

Find a route that includes water (river, sea or lake). Dr Martin Mau – who studies transformational distance hikes – told me that water is frequently cited in interviews as being 'of significance'.[11]

"Walks where we don't know what lies around the corner spark our imagination"

Meanwhile, Dutch environmental psychologists have identified spaciousness as conducive to a loss of self and ego, and to a radically raised mood. 'Our studies show that people feel less anxious and stressed, more connected to the landscape, and less concerned with themselves in spacious environments,' said cognitive psychologist Thomas van Rompay. 'In particular anxiety seems to rise in very wild, dense landscapes bereft of any sign of humanity. For a more transcendent experience – by which I mean loss of self and ego alongside greater feelings of connection – open space appears to be important.'

To boot, Rompay suggests finding a landscape or route suffused with mystery. 'Walks where we don't know what lies around the corner or over the hill spark our imagination, providing the unpredictability that can nudge us into a state of flow.'[12]

Psychologists also think that periods of silence are an essential part of long-distance walking, helping us to facilitate an inner dialogue. If we are bombarded by low-flying aircraft, thundering juggernauts or leaf blowers, not only will our inner voice be blotted out, but raised levels of stress will make it impossible to transition into a state of flow. For this reason, a long-distance route should avoid arterial or busy roads. Old drovers' routes, bridleways, footpaths, quiet country lanes and well-trodden pilgrim routes are ideal – and in part because they offer opportunities to converse.

In fact, spending some time with others (praying, sharing a meal or simply talking) was traditionally a vital part of a pilgrimage. And while periods of silence might be essential for reflection, psychologists have found that relationships with other (unknown) pilgrims also provide therapeutic benefits. 'Stories are exchanged, and we may get close to others relatively quickly, by sharing our difficulties with "sympathetic strangers",' said a researcher, noting that the transience of these relationships often accelerated a sense of intimacy – which in itself played a part in the healing process. This 'shortcut' to intimacy among strangers has also been explored by Dutch psychologist Dr Paul van Lange, who refers to the phenomenon as Vitamin S. 'Most of our relationships include a power dynamic even if we're unaware of it. But two strangers are truly equal, and equally vulnerable. Besides, strangers are unlikely to spread private information because they aren't in your social network,' he told me.[13] Lara's experience bears this out: she returned from her walk with three new friends, saying, 'We became very close, very quickly, and, ten years on, we still meet regularly despite living across three continents.'

But what about the inevitable physical pain – the blisters, strained muscles and aching shoulders? Again, our biology comes to the rescue. On distance walks, pain is often blocked by the body's own pain relief – opioid peptides like endorphins and enkephalins, and an endocannabinoid known as anandamide, have been shown to mask pain and anxiety in mice doing endurance exercise.[14]

But don't be too hasty with the ice packs: psychologists think (mild) physical pain is a vital part of the existential nature of a distance walk. Some use the phrase 'the body as memorial' to demonstrate how pain can attain meaning while walking for hour upon hour, day after day. Here, ideas of our wounded psyche or soul are mirrored in the tangible wounds of our blistered feet and sweetly aching calves. Physical pain can 'serve as a vicarious expression of the psychological or emotional pain we might be feeling', explained Rompay. Yes, even your blisters can be cathartic.

And finally, in addition to easing our minds, long-distance walking also helps our bodies: lower blood pressure, enhanced immunity and weight loss have all been identified as physiological benefits,[15] as well as improved sleep.[16]

notes

Distancing oneself from landscapes we know can provide the opportunity to reflect from a different perspective, so try walking somewhere utterly unfamiliar. A 2009 study of transformative travel concluded that 'those who experienced the most significant transformation visited settings far removed from their home.'

If you usually walk by the sea, head for the mountains. If you live somewhere hilly, go somewhere flat.

Ideally, find a route that passes through diverse and varied landscapes.

Need silence but don't want to walk alone? Many organisations now offer silent pilgrimages. Alternatively, join a group and specify a time when you'll be walking silently. Walking in silence alongside others can, in my experience, be a very powerful experience.[17]

Routes that hold a delicate and thrilling balance between the marks of Homo sapiens and the intractable wildness of nature are a favourite of mine – from the ancient drovers' routes that cross the Welsh mountains to Spain's Lighthouse Way. Here, temporal and geographical spaces collide, giving us numerous opportunities for a renewed sense of perspective.

Don't like the sound of 'long-distance walking'? Professor Kip Redick describes the combination of distance walking and the flow state as 'spiritual rambling'.[18] Consider yourself a spiritual rambler . . .

Turn your phone off. In studies, researchers have noted how often walkers talked about the joy of escaping the smallness and modernity of screen technology, and escaping into the timeless, embodied spaces their ancestors once encountered.

Marriage or family falling apart? Consider a pilgrimage: When researchers surveyed couples and families walking Spain's Camino, they found that walking a pilgrim route 'helps to strengthen marital bonds and trust, improves communication and mutual connection, shows care and affection and improves contact with children'.[19]

Don't shy away from encounters with strangers. Not only do these appear to add to the healing element of a pilgrimage, but they might also expand our brains. Van Lange's studies have found that communicating with people we don't know activates often dormant neural networks, boosting our 'mental fitness'.[20]

Unsure where to start? Barry Stone's *1001 Walks You Must Experience Before You Die* and Lonely Planet's *Epic Hikes of Europe* are wonderful teasers. For guided (and silent) pilgrimages, try the British Pilgrimage Trust.

A 2024 study of the flow state using EEG concluded that, ultimately, flow is about letting go, about 'decreased activity in brain parts involved in executive control.'[21] Surrender, surrender, surrender.

Mountains

The (Hormonal)
Enchantments of Elevation

'The mountains are calling,
and I must go.'

JOHN MUIR, LETTER TO HIS SISTER

— — — — — — — —

DEFINITION: A high area of land that rises steeply
above its surroundings, larger than a hill and often with
a pointed top. In the British Isles, an elevation above
2,000 ft/ 610 m is classified as a mountain.*

BENEFITS FOR: Confusion, loss of perspective, sluggish
immunity, hubris, anxiety, depression, low mood.

---

* However, the United Nations Environment Programme classifies a
mountain as a landmass with a peak above 8,200 ft (2,500 m).

I n 1881 Lizzie Le Blond was barely out of her teens, a new mother to a son conceived on her honeymoon, and unhappily married. She took herself to Chamonix in the Alps, telling her family that she needed Alpine air to cure her troublesome lungs. But I suspect she also went in search of a cure for her mind, her mood and her unsatisfactory marriage.

From beneath the shadow of Mont Blanc, Lizzie began taking daily walks until, one day, she found herself two thirds of the way up Mont Blanc. No one knows what epiphany struck that day, but two years and many mountain hikes later (including scaling Mont Blanc twice), she wrote her first book, *The High Alps in Winter: Or, Mountaineering in Search of Health*. She went on to hike and climb thirty-five peaks of over 4,000 metres, many of them never previously attempted by a woman.

"The man who has been to the mountains is never the same again"

Lizzie's mountain hikes and climbs precipitated a complete life change. Instead of returning to motherhood and the social whirl of London, she became a writer, an accomplished medal-winning photographer, and one of the first women to make films. She also founded, and was president of, the Ladies' Alpine Club – all at a time when well-born women were expected to do little more than visit their dressmakers and organise dinner parties. The mountains had changed her forever, she explained in 1932, writing, 'I owe a supreme debt of gratitude to the mountains for knocking from me the shackles of conventionality.'

Lizzie isn't the only person to take a walk in the mountains and return utterly changed. The history of walking spills over with people recounting transformative experiences while hiking at altitude. 'The man who has been to the mountains is never the same again,' wrote Indian mountaineer Major Hari Pal Singh Ahluwalia, after a lifetime of climbing the Himalayas.[1]

"When we walk at altitude we are biochemically changed"

What is it about mountains that so profoundly affects us? Why are so many of us changed by this often demanding landscape? Scottish writer Nan Shepherd wondered if it was the 'rarer air', writing, 'I am a mountain lover because my body is at its best in the rarer air of the heights and communicates its elation to the mind.' But she also wondered whether it might be something to do with her eyes, which 'delight in the expanse of space'. Or, she mulled, was it 'the sustained rhythm of movement in a long climb?' Shepherd concluded that her love of mountains was rooted in something more mystical, less easily explainable.[2]

"Panoramic views calm us"

She was right. When we walk at altitude, with vast vistas at every turn, we are biochemically changed. And these subtle changes prime us for more profound experiences.

Mountains offer us height, from where we can look out across the great expanse of beyond. Our eyes find this inherently restful, switching from the tight focal vision we use for screens and scrolling, to panoramic or vista vision, whereby our eyes sweep over the horizon. This shift of vision immediately quietens feelings of anxiety and fear (neuroscientist Andrew Huberman describes this as 'turning off the stress response by changing the way that we view our environment'[3]), explaining why we humans love wide, generous views. Put simply, panoramic views calm us.[4]

But height and wide-ranging views also give us perspective. From our mountain elevation we look down on the material world. Not only are we ourselves dwarfed by the mountains and the limitless sky above, but the world we have so painstakingly created – buildings, roads, towns – has collapsed to almost nothing.

To see the things that make us feel overwhelmed and exhausted rendered miniscule and toy-like helps us make sense of our world and our place in it. Up on the mountain, we are temporarily outside of that world with its incumbent difficulties and demands. In the strenuousness of our climb we have reduced it to something manageable. Meanwhile, the mountain has revealed us as we are – ant-small, inconsequential.

This strange paradox – that we can look down on the paltry smallness of our overwhelming life while simultaneously rendered tiny by the landscape – makes us feel at once emboldened and humble, amplified and diminished. And so we often return from the mountains with a revised sense of perspective.

A version of this cognitive shift was experienced by astronauts for decades. Writer Frank White coined the term 'overview effect' to describe the altered perceptions of astronauts returning to Earth, having seen the planet as little more than an illuminated marble floating in infinity.*

"The higher participants climbed, the less depressed, anxious, confused or angry they felt"

Granted, we aren't exactly orbiting the planet as we hike a mountain. But the two share surprising similarities. For a few hours we escape the quotidian frenzy of our lives and we shrink, then zoom out, setting ourselves and the world into

---

* Many returned with a new eco-consciousness and feeling of connection to others, as well as a deep sense of purpose as guardians of our fragile planet. In the words of Edgar Mitchell (Apollo 14): an 'overwhelming sense of oneness and connectedness . . . accompanied by an ecstasy . . . an epiphany'.

radically altered proportions. Curiously, our perceived size is determined by the view. As the Portuguese poet Fernando Pessoa said, 'I am the size of what I see.'[5]

In 2022 a group of Korean scientists, intrigued by the findings of so many forest-bathing studies (see Chapter 1, 'Forests and Woodland'), asked whether 'green space' researchers might have overlooked something. Could altitude be modifying, altering or affecting the health benefits of forests? They set to work, sifting through dozens of studies to find those that included data on altitude. They then began picking apart the twenty-seven most robust studies, finding (as they had suspected) that the higher participants climbed, the less depressed, anxious, confused or angry they felt. This dramatic shift in mood was most marked during initial ascents to an altitude of 900 m, roughly the height of England's highest peak, Scafell Pike.[6]

"Our body produces more of a hormone called erythropoietin"

So why does our mood rise as we climb? Our own sense of self-esteem and pride? The additional feel-good biochemicals churning through us? These undoubtedly figure, but the researchers also noted that 'the thermal index (THI) and illuminance (lx) levels were significantly associated with the effect size of psychological restoration, suggesting that heat and light conditions are potential effect modifiers'. As we climb, the air cools and circulates more easily, making us feel more comfortable. But the light changes too – at altitude the light is less dense and less polluted, making it seem cleaner, brighter and sharper. Exactly the sort of light we humans love (see Chapter 10, 'Lakes' for more on why we love light).

Lastly, the researchers acknowledged that the sheer exertion involved in a long, sustained, uphill walk played a pivotal role in eradicating participants' feelings of anxiety. It's tempting to credit the hope molecules covered in the Introduction for the climbers' improved mood. But this is where things become interesting, because something else happens at altitude that scientists are just beginning to untangle. The higher we climb, the lower the atmospheric pressure, making it harder for the body to shift oxygen into the blood. To compensate, our body produces more of a hormone called erythropoietin (EPO), which, in turn, results in the production of more red blood cells. These enable oxygen to be shunted more efficiently round the body.

This isn't all that EPO can do. EPO also works on the central nervous system and appears to have antidepressant properties. In experiments, EPO has been found to rapidly lift the mood of participants, with effects that linger for a further three days.[7] When we hike at altitude, circulating EPO contributes to the brain-shifting and mood-lifting biochemicals coursing through our bodies. In fact, EPO also appears to have positive effects on our cognition, and this may be another reason that people living at moderate altitudes often live for longer and with less disease.

When I was midway through university (in the UK's flattest county), I too heard the call of the mountains. I needed height, distance, perspective, space. So I disappeared to the remote Himalayas, where I walked for three months and where whatever had broken gradually repaired itself. No one knew about EPO back then, but a few tests might have revealed my body to be awash in EPO.

EPO isn't the only biochemical that tests and biopsies would have thrown up. An examination of my blood and tissues would also have shown high quantities of active immune cells (natural killer cells and CD8T cells), thanks to the daily, arduous climbs – which are always part and parcel of a mountain hike.

When patients with Lynch syndrome (a genetic condition that can lead to cancer at a young age) exercised vigorously for forty-five minutes, oncologists noticed that the patients' immune systems were much more adept at stamping out cancer cells when compared to patients not exercising as much. They suspected the heart-pumping bouts of movement activated immune cells, which behave like a cancer-surveillance system, hunting down and destroying potentially cancerous cells. Think of our immune cells after a mountain climb as a bunch of dozing security guards suddenly given a double espresso and an intruder to waylay.

'The public should know that engaging in any form of exercise will somehow lead to effects in cancer prevention,' oncologist Eduardo Vilar-Sanchez told Medscape in 2023.[8]

More recently, the sort of exertion required to mountain climb has also been shown to reap benefits for our microbiome, with new studies indicating that 'huff and puff' results in greater diversity, abundance, resilience and versatility of mood-boosting and health-enhancing gut microbiota.[9] Even more intriguing, an extremely new study has found that moderate altitude (defined as 1,500–3,000 m) benefits our microbiome, reducing the numbers of 'bad' proteobacteria while increasing the numbers of good bacteria.[10] How so? No one knows, and more research will undoubtedly follow.

So Nan Shepherd was right – the 'expanse of space', 'the sustained rhythm of movement in a long climb', and the 'rarer air' neurochemically alter us. From this extraordinary, mysterious fusion of air, terrain and biochemistry, our minds are moved, our spirits lifted. And so Lizzie Le Blond was right too: mountain walking is medicine.

notes

A weekend is all it takes: a study of Alpine walking found positive effects on psychological resilience after a mere two days.[11]

Head for the heights: our bodies typically start to release EPO at elevations of 1,800 m and above, although we are all different and respond differently to altitude.[12]

Seek out tumbling mountain rivers and spend time beside them. One study found that mountain streams were perceived by walkers to be particularly 'beneficial to human health'.[13]

Wear sunscreen: Higher altitude means increased risk of sun-induced skin damage. UV radiation exposure increases 4 to 5 per cent with every 1,000 feet (300 m) above sea level. So at an altitude of 9,000 to 10,000 feet (2,750–3,050 m), UV radiation may be 35 to 45 per cent more intense, according to the Skin Cancer Foundation. Violet light is not all bad, however: new studies suggest the violet light – in moderation – can help prevent myopia and improve alertness, cognition and memory.

Keep your head up. The human head is heavy, and when walking uphill we can be tempted to let it fall forward. This can shift the alignment of our entire body, straining the shoulders, neck and back.

Lift your chest up and keep your shoulders wide and relaxed – this will make breathing feel easier.

It can be tempting to bend at the waist while moving uphill, but this too throws the body out of alignment. Try and stay as upright as possible, bending the ankles forward rather than the waist.

Swing your loosely bent arms as you walk. The additional momentum will help propel you upwards, as well as burning a few extra calories and encouraging blood to keep shunting round the body.

Alternatively, take a pair of walking poles, which will allow your upper body to bear some of the burden. Studies show that walking with poles reduces feelings of fatigue. They also help with balance on both ascents and descents.

Concerned about the sheer difficulty of a mountain climb? Don't be – doing things that require extreme effort and attention releases feel-good dopamine, while fostering a sense of agency, resilience and, according to pioneering mountaineer Henriette d'Angeville, 'spiritual wellbeing'. Reframe any perceived hardship as 'the kinaesthetic pleasures of one's body moving at the limit of its ability' (as Rebecca Solnit put it in *Wanderlust: A History of Walking*).

Note: Shepherd and Le Blond were never at extreme altitude, which can be detrimental to health and wellbeing for most of us. Look for moderate altitude – I like a height of between 1,000 and 3,000 metres.

Rivers

Our Primal Partners

'The stream invites us to follow: the impulse is so common that it might be set down as instinct; and certainly there is no more fascinating pastime than to keep company with a river.'

W. H. HUDSON, *AFOOT IN ENGLAND*

DEFINITION: A large, natural stream of water flowing in a channel to the sea, a lake, or another river.

BENEFITS FOR: Feeling lonely or in need of company; a frazzled mind in need of calm; craving reassurance when life becomes unpredictable.

n 2005, Li An Phoa was carefully filtering water from the River Rupert in Canada when she noticed a fellow canoeist eyeing her oddly. 'You won't need that thing here,' he said, 'you can drink straight from the river.' He knelt on the bank and began scooping handfuls of water straight into his mouth.

Li An's eyes filled with tears. 'I was born in the Dutch delta – the apotheosis of riverscapes – but it had never occurred to me that river water could be drunk like that,' she tells me. 'And yet that's exactly what our ancestors would have done. The moment was very emotional for me.' Within a few days of drinking nothing but river water, Li An noticed that her hair seemed thicker and claimed her eyesight was so improved she no longer needed to wear her glasses.

Three years later, Li An returned to walk the river. To her horror, its delicious, sweet waters were so polluted that the water was undrinkable. Wildlife had disappeared, poisoned by mercury. The people that once lived from its banks had been dispersed, pushed away by dams, hydroelectric plants, factories and commercial logging operations. 'I saw then that a clean river is a sign of a healthy economy, and I decided to devote my life to making rivers drinkable,' she explains.

Since then, Li An has walked over 18,500 km of river path, set up the Drinkable Rivers Foundation, delivered TED Talks, written a book and campaigned constantly for cleaner waters. 'Clean river water is good for our teeth, it's more easily digestible, it nourishes the microbiome in our gut and our mouth – and it tastes nothing like tap water,' she explains. 'When we drink clean water, it opens up our taste buds and improves the bacterial quality of our saliva.'

Like Li An, many of us are drawn to flowing water. Travel writing is rich with riverside walks, from Colin Thubron following the Amur River to Clara Vyvyan following the Rhône, from Anaïs Nin walking beside the Seine to Charles Dickens ambling along the River Thames. 'Nothing,' wrote John Cowper Powys in his memoir, compares 'to the pleasure I got when walking along the river's edge.' For D. H. Lawrence, a river was more than water: it was 'a form of extended consciousness'.

"Being near water seemed to kindle 'greater social connectedness'"

In one of the earliest indicators that flowing water affects our mental wellbeing, a team of American researchers studied sixty-seven veterans taking part in a four-day river trip organised by a charity called Rivers of Recovery. The researchers used a battery of tests to measure before and after levels of psychological stress among the participating veterans. They found significant improvements on every measure, not only immediately after the veterans' trip, but also a month later. PTSD symptoms had fallen by 19 per cent, stress symptoms had reduced by 28 per cent, sleep quality had improved by 11 per cent, depression had reduced by 44 per cent and anxiety by 31 per cent. The veterans reported feeling considerably calmer, confident and more positive.[1]

A few years later, another team of researchers decided to dig a little deeper into the mounting evidence that water could lift mood and raise spirits. This time, the researchers pulled together all the fledgling data on 'blue space'. After assessing thirty-three studies, they concluded that spending time near water 'can have direct benefit for health, especially mental health and psycho-social wellbeing.' Their analysis revealed that most experiments into blue and green space had indeed found a positive association between the presence of water and health and wellbeing indicators. Interestingly, they also noticed that being near water seemed to kindle 'greater social connectedness' – a theme that was to appear again and again. The researchers called on governments, planners and developers to invest in blue spaces, and on other researchers to investigate possible explanations for the effect of water on our minds.[2]

"People felt calmer and happier when walking alongside running water"

And yet much of the research into blue space lumped sea, rivers and lakes into a single amorphous mass. As we know, the ocean – or a lake, for that matter – bears little resemblance to a stream. Frustrated at this constant melding of very different blue spaces, a team of researchers from King's College London set up an experiment to study only the impact of rivers and canals. After all, for most urban dwellers, getting to the ocean or a lake is often impossible. What if rivers and canals – readily accessible in most towns and cities – could also transform our sense of wellbeing, they wondered.

Their study[3] involved a smartphone app where 300 participants logged their emotional states while walking beside rivers and canals over a period of fourteen days. Once again, the results suggested that being beside rivers and canals 'was associated with significantly higher levels of wellbeing'. People felt calmer and happier when walking alongside running water, an effect that was 'long-lasting'. The researchers also noted that 'compared to being anywhere else, participants were more likely to report feeling safe both during the day and (a little unexpectedly) at night, as well as feeling socially included when visiting canals and rivers'. Once again, blue space seemed to confer feelings of social connection, of being companioned – a feeling that endured even at night, when (presumably) the rivers and their banks were quiet and unpeopled.

Moreover, this study found that although rivers and canals had a positive effect on all respondents (regardless of age, mental health, gender and education), the effect was more marked on young people and on men. The King's College researchers scratched their heads, perplexed. 'Why [might] visits to canals and rivers bear greater mental health benefits than [visits to] green spaces?' they asked. Was it because of possible encounters with a wide 'range of wildlife, including fish, ducks, herons and other water-dwelling species' (now known to affect our mood, see Chapter 14, 'Ecotones')? The researchers had no answers, but urged GPs to include river walks in their nature prescriptions.

"A mountain stream had an immediate effect, lowering blood pressure but accelerating heart rate"

So what is it about walking a river that soothes our frayed nerves with such effortless speed? Evolutionary biologists maintain that the sight of water triggers ancient memories of survival. For our distant nomadic ancestors walking out of Africa carrying babies, pelts, cooking pots, a glimpse of water dazzle on the horizon meant survival. Fresh water meant not only the quenching of thirst, but cooler air, the possibility of fish, animals and plants to eat, the chance to cleanse.

This might explain why, when Swiss and Austrian researchers[4] investigated mountainscapes, they found that the presence of a mountain stream had an immediate effect, lowering blood pressure but accelerating heart rate. Again, the researchers were bemused: Was the presence of a (very noisy) tumbling mountain stream 'activating the cardiovascular system or increasing vitality?'

"Water has a calming, relaxing yet energizing effect"

The answer may lie in the amplified presence of negative air ions (an air molecule combined with a water molecule and so carrying an extra negative charge) that linger in the air surrounding waterfalls and fast-moving water. Studies have found faster heart rates at waterfall sites,[5] prompting scientists to ask whether rapidly flowing water energises us by accelerating the circulation of blood, oxygen and nutrients in our bodies. As the researchers summed up: 'Mountain rivers . . . seem to provide health benefits'.[6]

Another answer to the calming yet invigorating effects of water might lie in its colour. Of course, water isn't blue. But when it reflects the sky, it can appear blue, and neurosurgeon Amir Vokshoot thinks this might contribute to water's 'calming, relaxing yet energizing effect [which stimulates] a positive emotional response . . . related to the effects of dopamine'. We like blue, he adds, because we evolved on a planet comprising primarily of shades of blue.[7]

And yet not all rivers comfort and calm us. A growing body of evidence suggests that we have an inherent distaste for dirty, polluted water. We yearn not for any old flowing water, but for *clean* flowing water. Given the dangers of filthy water, not to mention the unsightliness, it's perhaps not surprising. But what startled researchers was the immediacy and speed with which people stopped visiting unclean rivers. When a group of scientists banded together to investigate Europe's waterbodies, they compared cleanliness (based on the EU's water-quality monitoring system) with number of visits. Their analysis showed that every one-point level of improvement in water quality resulted in 6.67 more visitors, while a one-level deterioration resulted in dramatically fewer visits (–21 per cent).[8]

Clean water is rich in minerals – calcium, potassium sodium, fluoride, iron. But it also reflects light, attracts fish, reptiles, birds and insects, feeds a wide diversity of plants, and acts as a natural community hub – whether of houseboats, anglers, rowers or simply other strollers. Few walks can surpass a river walk.

notes

New studies show that proximity to rivers, as well as lakes and oceans, can protect against heart attacks triggered by extreme temperature, thanks to water's molecular, heat-absorbing properties that keep the nearby land at a more moderate temperature. When temperatures soar or plunge, find a river and walk beside her.[9]

Take your children or grandchildren to the river as often as you can. New research across eighteen countries suggests that growing up with regular exposure to blue space is linked to a lower prevalence of mental health disorders in adulthood.[10]

Many river walkers – including Li An – have a preference for walking source to sea. But sometimes we like to go against the flow, like a salmon bravely swimming upstream. It feels, perhaps, a little more radical. Choose your direction according to your mood.

How long do we need to be beside a river for our minds to shift gear? Not long. When a team of environmental psychologists compared the effects of falling, flowing and still fresh water using EEG to monitor brainwaves, they found a mere three minutes was all it took for participants' brainwaves to switch into alpha mode – our most relaxed awake state.[11]

Pay special attention to the confluence of two rivers – these points were once considered spiritually significant, but today are acknowledged as points of ecological import. Confluence zones often have altered water speed, temperature and chemistry, attracting differing plant, bird and insect life.

And finally, for anyone sceptical that Li An's eyesight improved as a result of drinking clean river water, bear in mind that while clean water is rich in minerals (including zinc, thought to be essential for eyes), tap water is typically 'purified' of most nutrients. Always use a high-quality portable filter if you want to drink from rivers.

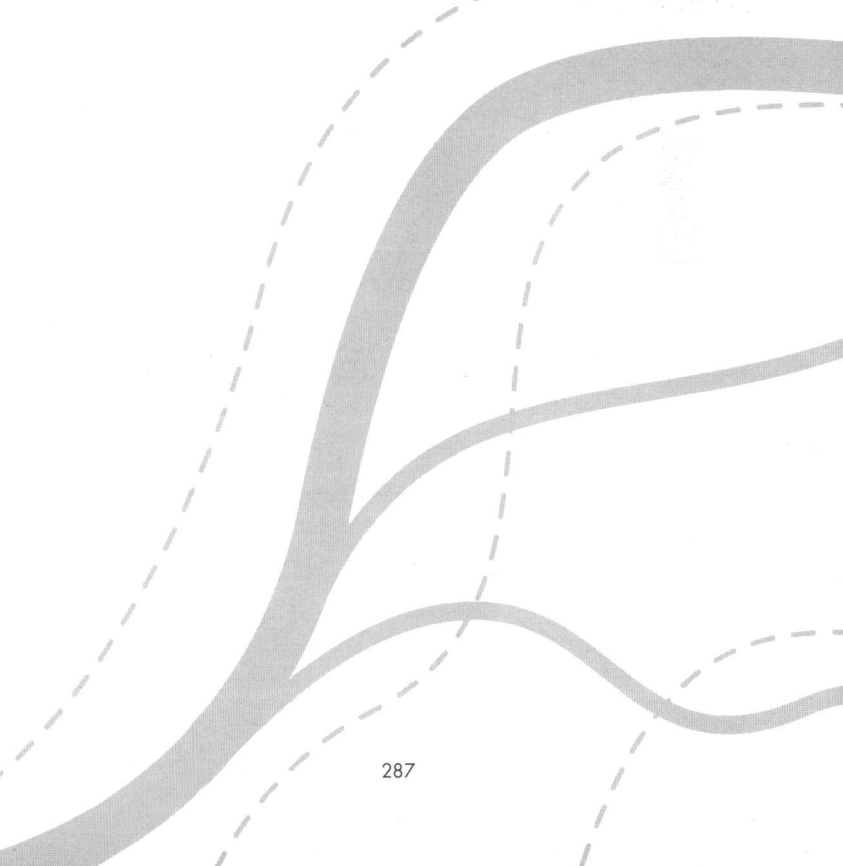

CHAPTER 20

Nocturne

The Neurochemical Nature
of Celestial Vaulting

'When we are chafed and fretted by small cares, a look at the stars will show us the littleness of our own interests.'

MARIA MITCHELL[1]

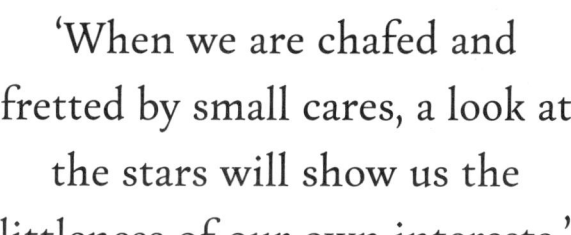

DEFINITION: From the Latin *nocturnus*, 'belonging to the night'. Used here to mean any landscape experienced in darkness.

BENEFITS FOR: Insomnia, rumination, boredom, sensory overload, feeling disconnected from our bodies and senses, feeling without purpose.

The artist Georgia O'Keeffe started night walking after arriving in Texas, aged twenty-four. Having grown up on a prairie farm, neither darkness nor unending space frightened her. Rather, they inspired her. And to the concerned friends who fretted for her safety, she replied, 'There is nothing to be afraid of – because there is nothing out there.'

O'Keeffe walked alone or sometimes with her sister, striding across the utterly black plains, her ears full of the cries of night-flying birds and the tumultuous winds that gusted over the arid, boundless Texas panhandle. 'I loved the starlight – the dark – the wind,' she wrote after one midnight walk. Again and again, O'Keeffe's letters talk of 'the emptiness of the night', the 'big quiet moonlight', the 'wonderful big starlight'. The dark intrigued her. Sometimes it seemed to accompany her, at other times it ignored her. Occasionally she sensed it chasing her, 'an enormous – intangible – awful thing'. In her more candid moments, however, O'Keeffe confessed to the fear she felt on these walks. 'I was afraid,' she wrote in a letter. 'Didn't say so – but I was – I was terribly afraid.'[2]

From this jostle of fear and exhilaration, O'Keeffe found inspiration. She began painting what she saw and felt in darkness – skies prickling with stars, wavering moons, empty indigo infinity. O'Keeffe isn't the first person to creep out for a night walk. Charles Dickens is well known for night walking:

following the death of his father, he spent many nights walking manically all over London, trying to outwalk his grief and his insomnia. Six years later, as his marriage crumbled, Dickens night walked again – this time getting up at 2 a.m. and walking 'over 30 miles – through the dead of night' to Kent. It was 'better to be up and doing something, than lying [in bed]', he wrote in a letter to a friend.

The artist Gwen John roamed the parks and suburbs of Paris after night, before rendering them in tiny watercolours. The writer Samuel Johnson pounded the streets of London with a friend, coining the term 'noctivagation', meaning 'the act of wandering in the night'. More recently, the writer Robert MacFarlane hijacked the term 'noctambulate' – a word that once meant 'to sleep-walk'.

As I researched a previous book,[3] I walked some of O'Keeffe's favourite nocturnal routes in the middle of the night. But it was to take me several more years before I felt comfortable walking alone in the dark. One winter, grieving a series of unexpected deaths and unable to sleep, I began getting up, dragging on boots and coat, and heading out over the open fields that surrounded my home. Action, I decided, was the antidote to grief. I wasn't as bold as Charles Dickens, but I was a little bolder than the Brontë sisters, who spent their grieving nights circumnavigating the kitchen table.

As time passed, I walked more and more at night, joining guided night hikes in the countryside, walking with friends in darkened cities, dragging my family through pitch-black forests and yomping alone in pursuit of moths, glow worms and meteorites. Night is a landscape like no other. And night walks are now among my favourite ways to move, particularly when I cannot sleep.[4]

As I mentioned in the Introduction, safety is (for me) one of the single most important requirements of a landscape. And yet this is why night walks are so thrilling, and why I'm including the 'landscape' of night. As we tell ourselves that we're completely safe (after all, wolves and highwaymen are long gone and no attacker would choose to lurk in a wet field at 3 a.m.), our brain tells us something else altogether.

We've evolved to be diurnal creatures – without visual stimuli, we can become tense and anxious.[5] Our brains begin pumping out corticotropin-releasing hormone. This hormone is responsible for co-ordinating our entire defence system, prompting the pituitary gland to release another hormone (called adrenocorticotropic hormone), which races through the blood to our adrenal glands, where the stress hormone, cortisol, is made. A sudden rush of cortisol gives us the energy we need to escape – fast!

"Our ears open, our nostrils sharpen, our sense of proprioception becomes more acute"

But here's the really interesting thing: new studies suggest that small doses of corticotropin-releasing hormone could have therapeutic benefits for both body and mind.[6] Some biologists think that micro-doses could be antidepressant and anti-cancerous. Why? Because the side effects of corticotropin-releasing hormone include a burst of anti-inflammatory glucocorticoids[7] and enhanced memory. Our sharpened brains work overtime to lay down memories of anything that might jeopardise our survival – including a pigeon flapping out of a tree and startling us as we walk. For the night stroller, this often means a vividly recalled walk.

"On night walks we are more animal and less human"

"When our sight is impeded, our body compensates"

Meanwhile, when our sight is impeded, our body compensates in several ways. Firstly, our weakly straining eyes prompt our brain and body to become hyper-alert and vigilant. Our ears open, our nostrils sharpen, our sense of proprioception becomes more acute. On night walks we are, of necessity, more animal and less human. We are more sensitive to smells. Our ears pick out the smallest of sounds. We are intensely aware of the terrain beneath the soles of our feet. We startle at a branch brushing against our skin. All of this is magnified in locations we don't know.

"In these quiet, calm moments we experience the magical qualities of nocturne"

Because we're in a heightened state of vigilance and acutely focused on the placing of our feet, we cease our ruminations.

Our brain cannot afford to expend valuable resources on ruminating when it needs to keep us safe from age-old fears – falling, drowning, fire, predators. And so night walks are utterly immersive and powerfully mindful.

As our eyes adapt to the low light, and as we become habituated to the dark, our fears fade – at least until the next time we hear rustling bushes or the screech of an owl. And in these quiet, calm moments we experience the magical qualities of nocturne – the night perfumes, the silence, the strange sense of having the world to oneself, the altered landscape in which we see only the rims and edges of things. A little surprisingly, all this is deeply calming.

At night we are exposed to experiences unavailable to us during the day – from plants that produce moth-attracting scents, to insects that only reveal themselves after dark, to the startling sounds of owls and night-migrating birds, to our own nocturnally altered brain. We may feel sensorily deprived – but this couldn't be further from the truth. Although there are none of the usual colour-saturated vistas and views, we can hear, sense and smell things that we overlook during the day.

Moreover, awe researchers (yes, they exist!) have found the night sky to be one of the most impressive sources of awe, wonder, enchantment – call it what you will. Science writer Jo Marchant refers to the experience of gazing upwards on a clear night as 'celestial vaulting'. We stare into the heavens and feel microscopically small. The light streaming from stars millions of miles away and the dazzling confluence of so much space and time renders us awe-struck and utterly enchanted, so that our own minuscule problems suddenly seem exactly that . . . minuscule.

"Darkness itself helps heal the body and mind"

But why so calming? According to science writer Florence Williams, feelings of awe manifest in physiological responses: 'A heightened awe experience stimulates the vagus nerve, which calms us, and releases a pleasant rush of dopamine and oxytocin, increasing a sense of connection,' she wrote in *Outside* magazine. 'It also dramatically shifts which brain networks are firing up.'[8] Brain scans show that feelings of awe lead to a less active default-mode network (the brain regions which turn on when we're daydreaming, often characterised as being 'inward-looking' and ruminative). Studies show that the awe-struck human not only feels a diminished sense of ego and self, but they're also more inclined to behave altruistically. Awe takes us out of ourselves.

Hot-off-the-press research now indicates that darkness itself helps heal the body and mind. As much as we need bright light during the day, and especially in the morning (see Chapter 10, 'Lakes'), so we also need dense, inky darkness at night. When researchers analysed data on light, dark, physical activity and mental health from the records of over 86,000 people, they found that those who spent six to eight hours in complete darkness at night were less likely to suffer from major depressive disorder, generalised anxiety disorder, PTSD, psychosis, bipolar disorder, and self-harm behaviour. 'We evolved to spend our nights in darkness and our days in light', explained Professor Sean Cain, an expert in circadian rhythms. 'Humans today challenge this biology, spending around 90 per cent of the day indoors under electric lighting, which is too dim during the day and too bright at night compared to natural light and dark cycles. It's confusing our bodies and making us unwell.'[9]

When we fail to get enough light during the day and enough darkness at night, we disrupt our delicate circadian rhythms in ways still not fully understood. As Cain told me, we need the healing power of darkness as much as we need the therapeutic qualities of light. Nor is this the first time that darkness has been linked to better mental health. Earlier studies found that 'dark therapy' – a term used for light-free nights – effectively reduced mania.[10]

In 2024 the psychologist Christopher Barnes devised a measurement for assessing our relationship with night, called the Night Sky Connectedness Index.[11] He had noticed that the surge of studies on nature and its benefits had overlooked the night sky. 'We seem to have become disconnected from the night,' he told me. 'This matters because, like the better known "green space", the night sky also has significant benefits for our mental health and happiness.'

"Darkness is a deeply tranquil and restorative experience"

Barnes's own interest was kindled during the pandemic, when he bought himself a telescope and began looking upwards. 'The idea was to have a little fun with my children, but as I watched YouTube videos on telescopes and astrophotography,

I noticed something about the language ... the YouTubers seemed to be experiencing something very special and deeply connecting when out at night.' Barnes began exploring the literature, then interviewing other night sky aficionados. And yet Barnes thinks more is at play than just awe.

"Having a connection to the night sky is important to our wellbeing"

'For me, and those I've listened to,' he explains, 'being in a place where you feel comfortable with the darkness is a deeply tranquil and restorative experience. It can bring a sense of peace and quiet contemplation. Yes, it can be cold and cloudy, but there's often a point when we lose ourselves and become absorbed by our surroundings, which is incredibly calming.'

Barnes's research also suggests that many of us feel reassured by the predictability of the constellations, planets and moon. 'Some of the people I interviewed referred to the celestial objects as old friends,' he added. 'The return of certain stars, planets and constellations was often a source of joy. For me, this speaks of a sense of place and purpose within our wider universe, and generally in life. Ultimately, I think that having a connection to the night sky is important for our wellbeing because of what it gives us – a place to be restored, inspired and free.'[12]

notes

If you decide to walk having been asleep for an hour or more, your eyes will already be dark-adapted — as long as you get dressed in either darkness or very low light. So don't turn on lights before you head off.

If you've had lights on, turn them off and sit in the dark for at least twenty minutes, which will allow your rods to adjust and start working.

Alternatively, leave at dusk and let your rods and cones adapt as the light falls naturally.

Blue light destroys night vision, so don't come straight from a fully glaring laptop either. And keep your phone turned off or on red mode.*

Full-moon nights mean we can walk without torches or headlamps, and with a greater sense of safety. These are my favourite nights for walking.

---

* Android users may need to download a red light app.

Walk your route by day first. Identify key waymarks that can be recognised by outline and shape rather than colour. Places can look very different by night, and it's much easier to become disorientated and lose our way when we can only see dimly.

Try walking on a windy night. In darkness, wind becomes – as O'Keeffe noticed – quite a different beast. Instead of being a minor nuisance, we feel acutely its brush against our skin; we notice the different sounds it makes as it blows through the branches of trees or ripples over grass; we sniff the odours carried from far-off farms.

Light and sound travel more readily at night. You'll hear the rip and tear of motorbikes from miles away, and spot the distant lights of far-flung houses. Marvel at the fact that while your vista is restricted, sounds, smells and splinters of light come to you from far away – an alchemy of sorts.

We smell more acutely after nightfall, with our olfactory bulb at its most sensitive around 9 p.m.[13] Take advantage of this by sniffing regularly, particularly after rainfall and in warm temperatures.

It's not just that our olfactory bulb is more efficient: smells can amplify in darkness. Why? Because during the day, the sun warms the earth, causing evaporation that creates an upward flow of water vapour, taking smells away. At night the ground cools, causing odours to diffuse horizontally. The smells are caused by bacteria that bind to water droplets and will be more pronounced after a downpour or in humid climates, for example.

Don't forget to look up. A clear night sky, replete with stars and planets, can induce a sense of reverence and wonder that reminds us of our (tiny) place in the world.

Uninspired by the stars? Take a UV torch and examine the way in which dozens of biofluorescent plants, insects, fungi, lichens (and more) change colour beneath its beam. For guided biofluorescent walks, try revealnature.co.uk

Go alone if you feel safe. According to Dr Barnes, 'most people like to be by themselves because there's a positive sort of solitude that we can rarely grab in the usual hubbub of life'.[14]

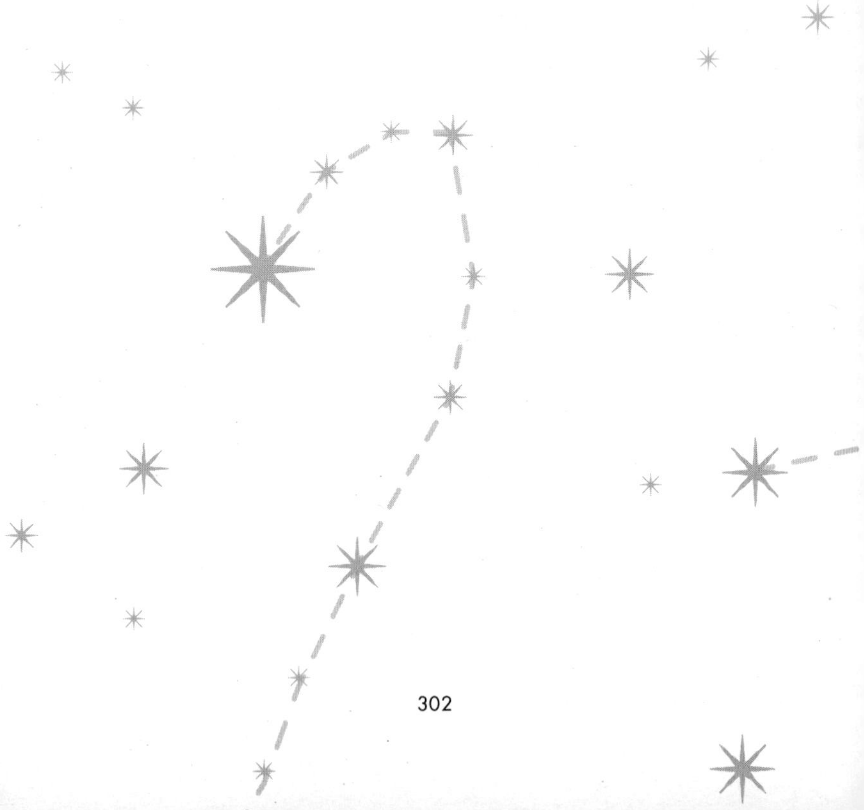

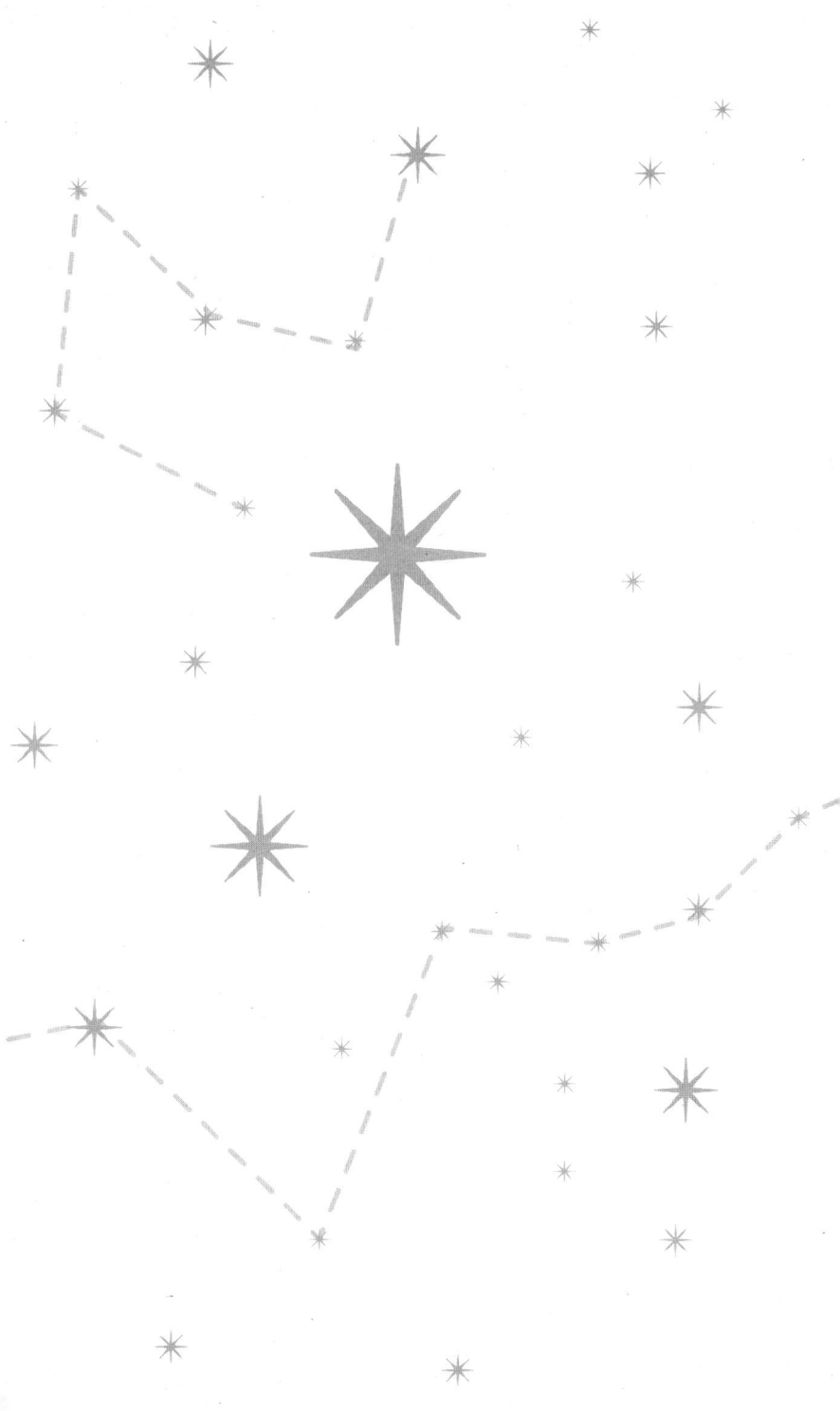

Epilogue

In this book, I've attempted to explore some of the fascinating neurochemical and biochemical alterations that strike in different landscapes. One of the most astonishing discoveries of the past year is that merely walking among trees and plants changes us at a cellular level by lengthening our telomeres, the repeating sections of DNA that sit at the end of each chromosome, preventing them from fraying and shortening. The great outdoors, it appears, can help us live with greater happiness and serenity, in better health, and for longer. Good, right?

And yet a growing body of evidence suggests that too much human presence in wild places (and in urban places, for that matter) is threatening landscapes, wildlife, air and water quality, even old buildings. A night walk or a mountain amble may be wonderful, life-enhancing experiences, but if all of us were to begin regularly night hiking and mountain climbing, there would be terrible repercussions for nocturnal animals and fragile mountain terrains. Meanwhile, driving polluting cars in order to inhale the clean air of a lake, or tossing our single-use water bottles into the trash after a seaside amble, merely contribute to the poor air and dirty water from which we are (temporarily) fleeing.

Tread lightly and reverently, go when you are called (but not every day), give as you have taken and understand that nature does not exist to serve our health and wellbeing. Lobby your town councils, planners and Members of Parliament for greener towns and cities, for more pedestrian routes, for non-polluting public transport. Press for more open space and trees, for cleaner rivers and purer air, and for the continued protection and preservation of the spaces and buildings that enchant and delight. We have never needed these as urgently as we do now.

Together, we can preserve our beautiful natural landscapes and create genuinely walkable cities. Together we can walk into a better preserved, less polluted, more diverse and ecologically resilient future. Together we can create cities that are safely and pleasurably walkable for everyone. For surely everyone deserves a joyfully walkable route from their own front door?

Acknowledgements

Many psychologists, researchers, scientists and writers helped in the production of this book, sending me papers and answering my questions. In no particular order, I'd like to thank Dr Amy McDonnell, Dr Christopher Barnes, Dr Sarah McKay, Dr Sharon Blackie, Sarah Wilson, Dr Catherine Kelly, Dr Michael Moore, Dr Lu Qi, Peter Ross, Clare Pooley, Sarah O'Hara, Dr Eamon Laird, Noreen Masud, Dr Ali Foxon, Dr Craig McDougall, Dr Megan Grace, Dr Fritz Gotz, Tim Evans, Emma Robertshaw, Jini Reddy, Dr Claire Nolan, Jo Bell, Jonathan Davidson, Duncan Minshull, Nick Hunt, Dr Thomas van Rompay, Dr Martin Mau, Li An Phoa, Professor Sean Cain, Dr Guy Hayward, Dr Katarina Borer, Dr Paul van Lange and David Atthowe. A huge thank you to everyone who so generously shared their walking stories with me over the last decade and to all the Age Well Project readers who took the time to answer my questions on landscape, space and place. Thank you – as ever – to Matthew, always my first reader, and to my mother, who raised me to be forever on foot. Last but not least, thank you to all my friends and family who regularly walk beside me: you know who you are!

Without the wonderful team at Bloomsbury and my dedicated, hard-working agents at Rachel Mills Literary, *The Walking Cure* would never have become a book: thank you to Rowan Yapp, Kate Quarry, Lauren Whybrow, Faye Robinson, Clare Baggaley, Victoria Denne, David Atkinson, Rachel Mills, Alexandra Cliff and Charlotte Bowerman. Keep walking!

Thank you, also, to: Nine Arches Press for kindly allowing me to quote from 'Lifted', included in *Kith* by Jo Bell (2015); Headline Publishing for kindly allowing me to quote from *A Tomb with a View* by Peter Ross (2020); Atlantic Books for kindly allowing me to quote from *Wild by Nature* (2014) by Sarah Marquis.

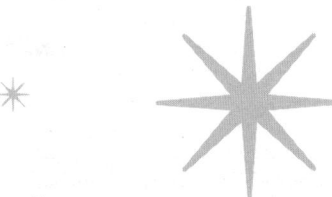

Notes

AUTHOR'S NOTE

1   L. Menatti and A. Casado da Rocha, 'Landscape and Health: Connecting psychology, aesthetics, and philosophy through the concept of affordance', *Frontiers in Psychology*, vol 7, 3 May 2016.

INTRODUCTION

1   B. Q. Ford, et al., 'The psychological health benefits of accepting negative emotions and thoughts: Laboratory, diary, and longitudinal evidence', *J. Pers. Soc. Psychol.*, 115(6), 2018, pp. 1075–92. DOI: 10.1037/pspp0000157

2   S. Blackie, *If Women Rose Rooted: A life-changing journey to authenticity and belonging*, September Publishing, 2016.

3   S. Wilson, *This One Wild and Precious Life*, Eye & Lightning Books, 2023.

4   B. Opitz, et al., *Places That Make Us*, National Trust and University of Surrey, 2017, with a 2019 follow-up study.

5   M. R. Marselle, et al., 'Moving beyond Green: Exploring the Relationship of Environment Type and Indicators of Perceived Environmental Quality on Emotional Well-Being following Group Walks', *Int. J. Environ. Res. Public Health*, 12(1), 2015, pp. 106–30, DOI: 10.3390/ijerph120100106

6   J. Barton and J. Pretty, 'What is the best dose of nature and green exercise for improving mental health? A multi-study analysis', *Environ. Sci. Technol.*, 44, 2010, pp. 3947–55.

7   D. Martens, et al., 'Walking in "wild" and "tended" urban forests: The impact on psychological well-being', *J. Environ. Psychol.*, 31, 2011, pp. 36–44.

8   M. R. Marselle, et al., 'Walking for well-being: Are group walks in certain types of natural environments better for well-being than group walks in urban environments?', *Int. J. Environ. Res. Public Health*, 10, pp. 5603–28.

9   G. Brancato, et al., 'Simulated nature walks improve psychological well-being along a natural to urban continuum', *J. Environ. Psychol.*, vol 81, June 2022, www.sciencedirect.com /science/article/abs/pii/S027249442200024X

10 See for example, M. Dallimer, et al., 'Biodiversity and the feel-good factor: Understand associations between self-reports human well-being and species richness', *BioScience*, 62, 2012, pp. 47–55.

11 M. R. Marselle, et al., 'Moving beyond Green'.

12 Email correspondence with author following blog post from Dr McKay, 14 February 2024.

13 The term 'hope molecule' was coined by a pair of researchers, after reporting on a rodent experiment in which mice denied exercise seemed to 'lose hope' and give up. 'Is there a "hope" molecule?' they asked. C. Phillips and A. Salehi, 'A Special Regenerative Rehabilitation and Genomics Letter: Is There a "Hope" Molecule?', *Physical Therapy*, vol. 96, issue 4, 1 April 2016, pp. 581–3, academic.oup.com/ptj/article/96/4/581/2686531

14 A. Marques, et al., 'Bidirectional Association between Physical Activity and Dopamine Across Adulthood: A Systematic Review', *Brain Sci.*, 11(7), 23 June 2021, p. 829. DOI: 10.3390/brainsci11070829

15 J. C. Basso and W. A. Suzuki, 'The Effects of Acute Exercise on Mood, Cognition, Neurophysiology, and Neurochemical Pathways: A Review', *Brain Plast.*, 2(2), 28 March 2017, pp. 127–52. DOI: 10.3233/BPL-160040

16 Ibid.

17 S. Lee, et al., 'Physiological significance of elevated levels of lactate by exercise training in the brain and body', *J. Biosci. Bioeng.*, 135(3), March 2023, pp. 167–75. DOI: 10.1016/ j.jbiosc.2022.12.001

18 J. Wang, et al., 'HSPA12A controls cerebral lactate homeostasis to maintain hippocampal neurogenesis and mood stabilization', *Transl. Psychiatry*, 13, 2023, p. 280. DOI: 10.1038 /s41398-023-02573-5

19 H. Han, et al., 'Exercise improves cognitive dysfunction and neuroinflammation in mice through Histone H3 lactylation in microglia', *Immun. Ageing*, 20(63), 2023. DOI: 10.1186/s12979-023-00390-4; immunityageing.biomedcentral.com/articles/10.1186/ s12979-023-00390-4

20 L. Gadye, 'A Secret in the Blood: How PF4 Restores Youth to Old Brains', University of California San Francisco Research, 16 August 2023, www.ucsf.edu/news/2023/08/4259 81/secret-blood-how-pf4-restores-youth-old-brains

21 N. Joisten, et al., 'Acute exercise increases systemic kynurenine pathway metabolites and activates the AHR in human PBMCs', bioRxiv, January 2024, DOI: 10.1101/2024.01.17. 576018

22 S. Brand, et al., 'Acute Bouts of Exercising Improved Mood, Rumination and Social Interaction in Inpatients with Mental Disorders', *Front. Psychol.*, 9:249, March 2018, DOI: 10.3389/fpsyg.2018.00249. And, for example, Y. Liu, et al., 'Physical activity and depression of Chinese college students: chain mediating role of rumination and anxiety', *Front. Psychol.*, 14:1190836, 31 July 2023. DOI: 10.3389/fpsyg.2023.1190836

23 G. Reynolds, 'The best treatment for depression? It could be exercise', *Washington Post*, 15 March 2023.

24 For more on how exerkines can 'frame' our perceptions, see Dr K. McGonigal's *The Joy of Movement*, Avery, 2019.

25 E. Kim, et al., 'Is altitude a determinant of the health benefits of nature exposure? A systematic review and meta-analysis', *Front. Public Health*, 25 November 2022, www.frontiersin.org/articles/10.3389/fpubh.2022.1021618/full

26 S. Park, et al., 'What Activities in Forests Are Beneficial for Human Health? A Systematic Review', *Int. J. Environ. Res. Public Health*, 19(5), 25 February 2022, p. 2692. DOI: 10.3390/ijerph19052692

27 S. Cao, et al., 'Cloudy or sunny? Effects of different environmental types of urban green spaces on public physiological and psychological health under two weather conditions', *Front. Public Health*, 28;11:1258848, 28 August 2023. DOI: 10.3389/fpubh.2023.1258848

28 J. Shi, et al., 'Contributions of residential traffic noise to depression and mental wellbeing in Hong Kong: A prospective cohort study', *Environ. Pollut.*, 338:122641, 1 December 2023. DOI: 10.1016/j.envpol.2023.122641

29 S. Blackie, *If Women Rose Rooted*, p. 339.

30 A. T. Gloster, et al., 'The spatiotemporal movement of patients in and out of a psychiatric hospital: an observational GPS study', *BMC Psychiatry*, 21, 2021, p. 165 DOI: 10.1186/s12888-021-03147-9

31 V. Sallay, et al., 'Profiles of perceived physical features and emotional experiences in favourite places: discovering ambivalent place preferences', *Journal of Environmental Psychology*, 90(4):102084, July 2023, DOI: 10.1016/j.jenvp.2023.102084

32 U. K. Stigsdotter, et al., 'Forest design for mental health promotion: Using perceived sensory dimensions to elicit restorative responses', *Landscape and Urban Planning*, vol. 160, April 2017, pp. 1–15, www.sciencedirect.com/science/article/pii/S0169204616302663

33 I. Otamendi-Urroz, et al., 'The role of emotions in human–nature connectedness within Mediterranean landscapes in Spain', *Sustain Sci.*, 18, 2003, pp. 2181–97, DOI: 10.1007/s11625-023-01343-y

34 E. Laird, et al., 'Physical Activity Dose and Depression in a Cohort of Older Adults in The Irish Longitudinal Study on Ageing', *JAMA Netw. Open*, 6(7):e2322489, 2023. DOI: 10.1001/jamanetworkopen.2023.22489

35 M. P. White, et al., 'Spending at least 120 minutes a week in nature is associated with good health and wellbeing', *Sci. Rep.*, 9, 7730 (2019). DOI: 10.1038/s41598-019-44097-3

36 For more on this subject, see Good Nature by K. Willis, Bloomsbury, 2024.

37 D. Matei, et al., 'The Endocannabinoid System and Physical Exercise', *Int. J. Mol. Sci.*, 24(3), 1989, 19 January 2023. DOI: 10.3390/ijms24031989

38 F. Fayet-Moore and S. R Robinson, 'A Breath of Fresh Air: Perspectives on Inhaled Nutrients and Bacteria to Improve Human Health', *Advances in Nutrition*, vol. 15, issue 12, 2024. DOI: 10.1016/j.advnut.2024.100333

1: FORESTS AND WOODLAND

1 All Carr quotes from E. Carr, *Hundreds and Thousands* (1927–41).

2 M. Tippett, 'Emily Carr's Forest', *Journal of Forest History*, vol. 18, issue 4, 1974, pp. 133–7. DOI: 10.2307/3983325

3 L. van Beethoven, *Beethoven: The Man and the Artist, as Revealed in His Own Words*, published in English by B. W. Huebsch, 1905, www.gutenberg.org/files/3528/3528-h/3528-h.htm

4 Q. Li, 'Effects of forest environment (Shinrin-yoku/Forest bathing) on health promotion and disease prevention – the Establishment of "Forest Medicine"', *Environmental Health and Preventive Medicine*, vol. 27, 2022, p. 43. DOI: 10.1265/ehpm.22-00160

5 Q. Li, et al., 'Effects of forest bathing (shinrin-yoku) on serotonin in serum, depressive symptoms and subjective sleep quality in middle-aged males', *Environ. Health Prev. Med.*, 27:44, 2022. DOI: 10.1265/ehpm.22-00136

6 Q. Li, 'Effects of forest environment'.

7 Q. Li, et al., 'Effects of forest bathing (shinrin-yoku) on serotonin'.

8 Y. Wen, et al., 'The Effects of Dynamic and Static Forest Bathing (Shinrin-yoku) on Physiological and Psychological Health in Males and Females', *Forests* 14, 2023, p. 1592. DOI: 10.3390/f14081592

9 J. Simkin, et al., 'Restorative effects of mature and young commercial forests, pristine old-growth forest and urban recreation forest: a field experiment', *Urban For Urban Green*, 48:126567, 2022. DOI: 10.1016/j.ufug.2019.126567

10 U. K. Stigsdotter, et al., 'Forest design for mental health promotion: Using perceived sensory dimensions to elicit restorative responses', *Landscape and Urban Planning*, vol. 160, April 2017, pp. 1–15, www.sciencedirect.com/science/article/pii/S0169204616302663

11 S. López-Pousa, et al., 'Sense of Well-Being in Patients with Fibromyalgia: Aerobic Exercise Program in a Mature Forest: A Pilot Study', *Evid. Based. Complement. Alternat. Med.*, 2015:614783. DOI: 10.1155/2015/614783

12 D. Donelli, et al., 'Effects of Plant-Emitted Monoterpenes on Anxiety Symptoms: A Propensity-Matched Observational Cohort Study', *Int. J. Environ. Res. Public Health*, 20(4), 4 February 2023, p. 2773. DOI: 10.3390/ijerph20042773

13 A. M. Pálsdóttir, et al., 'The qualities of natural environments that support the rehabilitation process of individuals with stress-related mental disorder in nature-based rehabilitation', *Urban Forestry & Urban Greening*, vol. 29, 2918, pp. 312–21. DOI: 10.1016/j.ufug.2017.11.016

14 S. Sudimac and S. Kühn, 'A one-hour walk in nature reduces amygdala activity in women, but not in men', *Front. Psychol.*, 13:931905, 27 September 2022; DOI: 10.3389/fpsyg.2022.931905

15 For more on E. Carr's forest fear and how she utilised it as 'creative gasoline', see Chapter 12 of *Sleepless* by A. Abbs.

16 E. Morita, et al., 'A before and after comparison of the effects of forest walking on the sleep of a community-based sample of people with sleep complaints', *Biopsychosoc. Med.*, 5:13, 14 October 2011. DOI: 10.1186/1751-0759-5-13

17 E. Ratcliffe, 'Sound and Soundscape in Restorative Natural Environments: A Narrative Literature Review', *Front. Psychol.*, 12:570563, 26 April 2021. DOI: 10.3389/fpsyg.2021.570563

18 U. K. Stigsdotter, et al., 'Forest design for mental health promotion: Using perceived sensory dimensions to elicit restorative responses', *Landscape and Urban Planning*, vol. 160, April 2017, pp. 1–15, www.sciencedirect.com/science/article/pii/S0169204616302663

19 K. -W. An, et al., 'Effects of Forest Stand Density on Human's Physiophychological Changes', *Journal of the Faculty of Agriculture*, Kyushu University, vol. 49, 2004. DOI: 10.5109/4588

20 H. Walker, et al., *Natural Volatile Organic Compounds (NVOCs) Are Greater and More Diverse in UK Forests Compared with a Public Garden*, 3 January 2023, repository.derby.ac.uk/download/0e3e53aad21c1cf4fbddcd8db3b72487602ea5a6217e4308e5e8ee23f49da575/1777440/forests-14-00092.pdf

2: SHORELINES

1 Quoted in E. Hunt, 'Blue spaces: why time spent near water is the secret to happiness' *The Guardian*, 3 November 2019, www.theguardian.com/lifeandstyle/2019/nov/03/blue-space-living-near-water-good-secret-of-happiness

2 M. Georgiou, et al., 'Mechanisms of Impact of Blue Spaces on Human Health: A Systematic Literature Review and Meta-Analysis', *Int. J. Environ. Res. Public Health*, 18(5), 3 March 2021, p. 2486. DOI: 10.3390/ijerph18052486

3 M. P. White, et al., 'Blue space, health and well-being: A narrative overview and synthesis of potential benefits', *Environmental Research*, vol. 191, December 2020, www.sciencedirect.com/science/article/pii/S0013935120310665

4 M. Elkins, et al., 'A Controlled Trial of Long-Term Inhaled Hypertonic Saline in Patients', *New England Journal of Medicine*, vol. 354, issue 3, 19 January 2006.

5 E. Cascetta, et al., 'The Effects of Air Pollution, Sea Exposure and Altitude on COVID-19 Hospitalization Rates in Italy', *Int. J. Environ. Res. Public Health*, 18(2), 8 January 2021, p. 452. DOI: 10.3390/ijerph18020452

6 M. N. Moore, 'Do airborne biogenic chemicals interact with the PI3K/Akt/mTOR cell signalling pathway to benefit human health and wellbeing in rural and coastal environments?' *Environmental Research*, vol. 140, July 2015, pp. 65–75.

7 A. Tobío, et al., 'Yessotoxin, a Marine Toxin, Exhibits Anti-Allergic and Anti-Tumoural Activities Inhibiting Melanoma Tumour Growth in a Preclinical Model', *PLoS ONE*, 11(12), 2016: e0167572. DOI: 10.1371/journal.pone.0167572

8 B. W. Wheeler, et al., 'Does living by the coast improve health and wellbeing?' *Health & Place*, 2012; DOI: 10.1016/j.healthplace.2012.06.015

9 S. J. Geiger, et al., 'Coastal proximity and visits are associated with better health but may not buffer health inequalities', *Communications Earth & Environment*, 4(1), 2023. DOI: 10.1038/s43247-023-00818-1

10 M. N. Moore, 'Do airborne biogenic chemicals . . .', and email correspondence with author, 12 September 2023.

11 A. L. Pearson, et al., 'Effects of freshwater blue spaces may be beneficial for mental health: A first, ecological study in the North American Great Lakes region', *PLoS ONE*, 14(8), 2019: e0221977. DOI: 10.1371/journal.pone.0221977

12 T. M. Lejeune, et al., 'Mechanics and energetics of human locomotion on sand', *J. Exp. Biol.*, 201(Pt 13), July 1998, pp. 2071–80. DOI: 10.1242/jeb.201.13.2071

13 A. Voloshina, et al., 'Biomechanics and Energetics of Walking on Uneven Terrain', *J. Ex.p Biol.*, 216(21), 2013, pp. 3963–3970. DOI: 10.1242/jeb.081711

14 'How walking in nature can help wellbeing', National Trust, www.nationaltrust.org.uk/discover/nature/how-walking-in-nature-can-help-wellbeing

15 R. G. Alloway, et al., 'An Explanatory Study Investigating the Effects of Barefoot Running on Working Memory', *Perceptual and Motor Skills*, 122(22), 2016, pp. 432–43. DOI: 10.1177/0031512516640391

16 T. Kim, et al., 'Barefoot walking improves cognitive ability in adolescents', *Korean J. Physiol. Pharmacol.*, 28(4), 2024, pp. 295–302. DOI: 10.4196/kjpp.2024.28.4.295

17 G. Chevalier, 'The effect of grounding the human body on mood', *Psychol. Rep.*, 116(2), April 2015, pp. 534–42. DOI: 10.2466/06.PR0.116k21w5

18 G. Chevalier, et al., 'The Effects of Grounding (Earthing) on Bodyworkers' Pain and Overall Quality of Life: A Randomized Controlled Trial', *Explore* (NY), 15(3), May–June 2015, pp. 181–90. DOI: 10.1016/j.explore.2018.10.001

19 'Corticotrophin-releasing hormone', You and Your Hormones, May 2020, www.yourhormones.info/hormones/corticotrophin-releasing-hormone

20 H. J. Park, et al., 'The Effect of Earthing Mat on Stress-Induced Anxiety-like Behavior and Neuroendocrine Changes in the Rat', *Biomedicines*, 11(1), , 26 December 2022, p. 57. DOI: 10.3390/biomedicines11010057

21 G. Chevalier, et al., 'Earthing (grounding) the human body reduces blood viscosity – a major factor in cardiovascular disease', *J. Altern. Complement. Med.*, 19(2), Feb 2013, pp. 102–10. DOI: 10.1089/acm.2011.0820

22 T. Börger, et al., 'The value of blue-space recreation and perceived water quality across Europe: A contingent behaviour study', *Sci. Total Environ.*, 771:145597, 1 June 2021. DOI: 10.1016/j.scitotenv.2021.145597

23 K. Sokal and P. Sokal, 'Earthing the human body influences physiologic processes', *J. Altern. Complement. Med.*, 17(4), 2011, pp. 301–8.

24 W. Menigoz, et al., 'Integrative and lifestyle medicine strategies should include Earthing (Grounding): Review of research evidence and clinical observations', *EXPLORE*, 16(3), 2020, pp. 152–60. DOI: 10.1016/j.explore.2019.10.005

3: LEAFY LANES AND RURAL ROADS

1 E. Thomas, *The Icknield Way*, 1913.

2 Y. da Silva and L. Hendry, 'Why road verges are important habitats for wildflowers and animals', Natural History Museum, www.nhm.ac.uk/discover/why-road-verges-are-important-wildlife-habitats.html

3 D. Y. Ouédraogo, et al., 'Can linear transportation infrastructure verges constitute a habitat and/or a corridor for vertebrates in temperate ecosystems? A systematic review', *Environ. Evid.* 9(13), 2020. DOI: 10.1186/s13750-020-00196-7

4 M. Guszkowska, 'Wpływ ćwiczeń fizycznych na poziom leku i depresji oraz stany nastroju [Effects of exercise on anxiety, depression and mood]', *Psychiatr. Pol.*, 38(4), July–August 2004, pp. 611–20. Polish. PMID: 15518309

5 C. Ma, et al., 'The effect of rhythmic movement on physical and cognitive functions among cognitively healthy older adults: A systematic review and meta-analysis', *Arch. Gerontol. Geriatr.*, January 2023; 104:104837. DOI: 10.1016/j.arcger.2022.104837

6 Interview in *The Guardian*, July 2019, www.theguardian.com/lifeandstyle/2019/jul/28/its-a-superpower-how-walking-makes-us-healthier-happier-and-brainier

7 B. del Pozo Cruz, et al., 'Association of Daily Step Count and Intensity with Incident Dementia in 78 430 Adults Living in the UK', *JAMA Neurol.*, 79(10), 2022, pp. 1059–63. DOI: 10.1001/jamaneurol.2022.2672 and B. del Pozo Cruz, et al., 'Prospective Associations of Daily Step Counts and Intensity with Cancer and Cardiovascular Disease Incidence and Mortality and All-Cause Mortality', *JAMA Intern. Med.*, 182(11), 2022, pp. 1139–48. DOI: 10.1001/jamainternmed.2022.4000

8 J. S. Y. Chan, et al., 'Special Issue – Therapeutic Benefits of Physical Activity for Mood: A Systematic Review on the Effects of Exercise Intensity, Duration, and Modality', *J. Psychol.*, 153(1), 2019, pp. 102–25. DOI: 10.1080/00223980.2018.1470487

9 J. L. Medina, et al., 'Optimizing the Exercise Prescription for Depression: The Search for Biomarkers of Response', *Curr. Opin. Psychol.*, 4, 2015, pp. 43–7. DOI: 10.1016/j.copsyc.2015.02.003

10 A. Dinoff, et al., 'The Effect of Exercise Training on Resting Concentrations of Peripheral Brain-Derived Neurotrophic Factor (BDNF): A Meta-Analysis', *PLoS One*, 11(9), 22 Septembr 2016, e0163037. DOI: 10.1371/journal.pone.0163037

11 S. Aritake-Okada, et al., 'Diurnal repeated exercise promotes slow-wave activity and fast-sigma power during sleep with increase in body temperature: a human crossover trial', *J. Appl. Physiol. (1985)*, 127(1), 2019. DOI: 10.1152/japplphysiol.00765.2018

12 L. A. Carlson, et al., 'Influence of Exercise Time of Day on Salivary Melatonin Responses', *Int. J. Sports Physiol. Perform.*, 14(3), 2019, pp. 351–3

13 G. S. Passos, et al., 'Effects of moderate aerobic exercise training on chronic primary insomnia', *Sleep Med.*, 2011; 12(10): 1018–27.

14 D. Matei, et al., 'The Endocannabinoid System and Physical Exercise', *Int. J. Mol. Sci.*, 24(3), 19 January 2023, p. 1989. DOI: 10.3390/ijms24031989

15 W. L. McGee, et al., 'Music interventions for acquired brain injury', *Cochrane Database Syst. Rev.*, 2017; Issue 1. Art. No.: CD006787. DOI: 10.1002/14651858.CD006787.pub3. And L. R. Nascimento, et al., 'Walking training with cueing of cadence improves walking speed and stride length after stroke more than walking training alone: A systematic review', *. J Physiother.*, 61(1), 2015, pp. 10–15. DOI: 10.1016/j.jphys.2014.11.015

4: ROLLING HILLS

1 L. Palumbo, et al., 'Comparing Angular and Curved Shapes in Terms of Implicit Associations and Approach/Avoidance Responses', *PLoS ONE*, 10(10), 2015, e0140043. DOI: 10.1371/journal.pone.0140043

2 N. Tawil, et al., 'The contour effect: Differences in the aesthetic preference and stress response to photo-realistic living environments', *Front. Psychol.*, 13:933344, 1 December 2022. DOI: 10.3389/fpsyg.2022.933344

3 E. G. Chuquichambi, et al., 'How universal is preference for visual curvature? A systematic review and meta-analysis', *Ann. N. Y. Acad. Sci.*, 1518(1), December 2022, pp. 151–65. DOI: 10.1111/nyas.14919

4 K. May, *Enchantment: Awakening Wonder in an Exhausted Age*, Faber & Faber, 2023.

5 A. Han and J. Kim, 'A Study of Leisure Walking Intensity Levels on Mental Health and Health Perception of Older Adults', *Gerontol. Geriatr. Med.*, 7:2333721421999316, 27 February 2021. DOI: 10.1177/2333721421999316

6 S. G. Parada-Sánchez, et al., 'The Effects of Different Types of Exercise on Circulating Irisin Levels in Healthy Individuals and in People with Overweight, Metabolic Syndrome and Type 2 Diabetes', *Physiol. Res.*, 71(4), 31 August 2022, pp. 457–75. DOI: 10.33549/physiolres.934896

7 S. Brand, et al., 'Acute Bouts of Exercising Improved Mood, Rumination and Social Interaction in Inpatients With Mental Disorders', *Front. Psychol.*, 9, 13 March 2018, p. 249. DOI: 10.3389/fpsyg.2018.00249

8 'Exercises & Nutrition to Support Eye Health', Huberman Lab Neural Network, 28 June 2023, www.hubermanlab.com/newsletter/exercises-and-nutrition-to-support-eye-health

9   V. L. Tseng, et al., 'Association between Exercise Intensity and Glaucoma in the
    National Health and Nutrition Examination Survey', *Ophthalmol. Glaucoma.*, 3(5),
    September–October 2020, pp. 393–402. DIO: 10.1016/j.ogla.2020.06.001

10 C. Wu, et al., 'Spacious Environments Make Us Tolerant: The Role of Emotion and
    Metaphor', *International Journal of Environmental Research and Public Health*, 18, no. 19, 2021,
    10530. DOI: 10.3390/ijerph181910530

11 J. Meyers-Levy and J. Zhu, 'The Influence of Ceiling Height: The Effect of Priming on
    the Type of Processing That People Use,' *Journal of Consumer Research*, 34, 2007,
    assets.csom.umn.edu/assets/71190.pdf

12 G. Bachelard, *The Poetics of Space*, trans. Maria Jolas, Penguin, 2014, p. 222.

13 Z. Song, et al., 'Daily stair climbing, disease susceptibility, and risk of atherosclerotic
    cardiovascular disease: A prospective cohort study', *Atherosclerosis*, 15 September 2023,
    www.atherosclerosis-journal.com/article/S0021-9150(23)05221-8/fulltext and correspon-
    dence with author, 9 October 2023.

14 K. T. Borer, 'How to Suppress Mineral Loss and Stimulate Anabolism in Postmeno-
    pausal Bones with Appropriate Timing of Exercise and Nutrients', *Nutrients*, 16(6),
    7 March 2024, p. 759. DOI: 10.3390/nu16060759

15 G. Robb, *Cols and Passes*, Particular Books, 2016, p. 11.

16 S. A. Linkenauger, et al., 'Choosing efficient actions: Deciding where to walk', *PLoS One*,
    14(9), 26 September 2019, e0219729. DOI: 10.1371/journal.pone.0219729

17 Quoted in S. Pyrah, 'The nature cure: How time outdoors transforms our memory,
    locic and imagination', *The Guardian*, 27 November 2023, www.theguardian.com/
    lifeandstyle/2023/nov/27/the-nature-cure-how-time-outdoors-transforms-our-
    memory-imagination-and-logic

18 K. Loria, 'Aerobic exercise boosts testosterone levels', *Urology Times*, 6 December
    2016, www.hubermanlab.com/newsletter/exercises-and-nutrition-to-support-eye-
    health

5: CEMETERIES

1   N. Price, *The Heart of a Vagabond*, Museum Press, 1955, p. 33.

2   Letter from Charlotte to Emily Brontë, 2 September 1843.

3   P. Ouellette, et al., 'The monastery as a restorative environment', *Journal of Environmental
    Psychology*, vol. 25, issue 2, June 2005, pp. 175–88.

4   Y. Zappaterra, *Cities of the Dead*, Franes Lincoln, 2022, p. 1.

5 H. Nordh, et al., 'A peaceful place in the city: A qualitative study of restorative components of the cemetery', *Landscape and Urban Planning*, 167(5), June 2017. DOI: 10.1016/j.landurbplan.2017.06.004

6 European Cemeteries Route, Council of Europe, www.coe.int/en/web/cultural-routes/the-european-cemeteries-route

7 I. Kowarik, et al., 'Biodiversity functions of urban cemeteries', *Urban Forestry & Urban Greening*, vol. 19, 1 September 2016, pp. 68–78.

8 Ibid.

9 A. Agbaje, 'Longitudinal mediating effect of fat mass and lipids on sedentary time, light PA, and MVPA with inflammation in youth', *Journal of Clinical Endocrinology & Metabolism*, 13 June 2023. DOI: 10.1210/clinem/dgad354

10 E. Laird, et al., 'Physical Activity Dose and Depression in a Cohort of Older Adults in The Irish Longitudinal Study on Ageing', *JAMA Netw. Open.*, 6(7), 3 July 2023, e2322489. DOI: 10.1001/jamanetworkopen.2023.22489

6: FLOWERS AND MEADOWS

1 T. K. H. Fung, et al., 'Therapeutic Effect and Mechanisms of Essential Oils in Mood Disorders: Interaction between the Nervous and Respiratory Systems', *Int. J. Mol. Sci.*, 22, 2021, p. 4844. DOI: 10.3390/ijms22094844

2 Ibid.

3 C. C. Woo, et al., 'Overnight olfactory enrichment using an odorant diffuser improves memory and modifies the uncinate fasciculus in older adults', *Front. Neurosci.*, 17:1200448, 24 July 2023. DOI: 10.3389/fnins.2023.1200448

4 B. S. Yasgur, 'Inhaling Pleasant Scents During Sleep Tied to a Dramatic Boost in Cognition', Medscape, 8 August 2023, www.medscape.com/viewarticle/995295

5 M. Leon and C. C. Woo, 'Olfactory loss is a predisposing factor for depression, while olfactory enrichment is an effective treatment for depression', *Front. Neurosci.*, 16:1013363, 28 September 2022. DOI: 10.3389/fnins.2022.1013363

6 G. Filiz, et al., 'Olfactory bulb volume and cortical thickness evolve during sommelier training', *Human Brain Mapping*, 43, 2022. DOI: 10.1002/hbm.25809

7 C. C. Woo, et al., 'Overnight olfactory enrichment . . .', 24 July 2023.

8 H. Walker, et al., 'Natural Volatile Organic Compounds (NVOCs) are Greater and More Diverse in UK Forests Compared with a Public Garden', *Forests*, 2023, 14(92). DOI: 10.3390/f14010092

9 K. Wendin, et al., 'Odor Perception and Descriptions of Rose-Scented Geranium Pelargonium graveolens "Dr Westerlund", Sensory and Chemical Analyses', April 2023, www.researchgate.net/publication/370541325_Odor_Perception_and_Descriptions_of_Rose-Scented_Geranium_Pelargonium_graveolens_'Dr_Westerlund'_-_Sensory_and_Chemical_Analyses

10 A. Al-Ayash, et al., 'The influence of color on student emotion, heart rate, and performance in learning environments', 26 February 2015. DOI: 10.1002/col.21949

11 M. Elsadek and B. Liu, 'Effects of viewing flowering plants on employees' wellbeing in an office-like environment', *Indoor and Built Environment.*, 30(9), 2021 pp. 1429–40. DOI: 10.1177/1420326X20942572

12 J. Haviland-Jones, et al., 'An environmental approach to positive emotion: Flowers', *Evol. Psychol.*, 3, 2005, pp. 104–32. DOI: 10.1177/147470490500300109

13 See for example, Y. Guan, et al., 'Exploring the Relationship between Trichome and Terpene Chemistry in Chrysanthemum', *Plants* (Basel), 11(11), 26 May 2022, p. 1410. DOI: 10.3390/plants11111410

14 M. I. Roslund, et al., 'Biodiversity intervention enhances immune regulation and health-associated commensal microbiota among daycare children', *Science Advances*, 6(42), 2020. DOI: 10.1126/sciadv.aba2578

15 A. Ito, et al., '"Green odor" inhalation by rats down-regulates stress-induced increases in Fos expression in stress-related forebrain regions', *Neurosci. Res.*, 65(2), October 2019, pp. 166–74. DOI: 10.1016/j.neures.2009.06.012

7: CITY STROLLING

1 D. Burtan, et al., 'Nature benefits revisited: Differences in gait kinematics between nature and urban images disappear when image types are controlled for likeability', *PLOS ONE*, 27 August 2021, DOI: 10.1372/journal.pone.0256635

2 C. San Juan, et al., 'Restoration and the City: The Role of Public Urban Squares', *Front. Psychol.*, 8:2093, 7 December 2017. DOI: 10.3389/fpsyg.2017.02093

3 S. Wang, et al., 'Urban cultural heritage is mentally restorative: an experimental study based on multiple psychophysiological measures', *Front. Psychol.*, 14:1132052, 17 May 2023. DOI: 10.3389/fpsyg.2023.1132052

4 J. Bermudez, et al., 'Externally-induced meditative states: an exploratory fMRI study of architects' responses to contemplative architecture', *Frontiers of Architectural Research*, vol. 6, issue 2, June 2017, pp. 123–6.

5 J. Martínez-Soto, et al., 'Exploring the Links Between Biophilic and Restorative Qualities of Exterior and Interior Spaces in Leon, Guanajuato, Mexico', *Front. Psychol.*, 12:717116, 17 August 2021. DOI: 10.3389/fpsyg.2021.717116

6 B. Hepworth, *Carvings and Drawings*, Manchester City Art Gallery, 1951, section 6.

7 Perceived air pollution was the main cause of discomfort along urban routes, followed by noise – according to this report: C. Vert, et al., 'Physical and mental health effects of repeated short walks in a blue space environment: A randomised crossover study', Open Research Exeter, 30 June 2020, ore.exeter.ac.uk/repository/bitstream/handle/10871/121710/Manuscript_shortWalksBlueSpaces_ER-20-847_REVISION_clean.pdf?sequence=2

8 L. B. Bloom, 'Ranked: The 30 most walkable cities in the world, according to a new report', *Forbes*, 30 January 2024, www.forbes.com/sites/laurabegleybloom/2024/06/30/ranked-the-30-most-walkable-cities-in-the-world-according-to-a-new-report

9 H. Xie, et al., 'Affective disorder and brain alterations in children and adolescents exposed to outdoor air pollution', *Journal of Affective Disorders*, vol. 33, 15 June 2023, pp. 413–24. DOI: 10.1016/j.jad.2023.03.082

10 K. K. Lau, et al., 'Dynamic response of pedestrian thermal comfort under outdoor transient conditions', *Int. J. Biometeorol.*, 63(7), July 2018, pp. 979–89. DOI: 10.1007/s00484-019-01712-2

8: FLATLANDS

1 All quotes from Noreen Masud, *A Flat Place*, Penguin, 2023.

2 Recounted in A. Abbs, *Windswept: Why Women Walk*, John Murray, 2021.

3 P. Conway, *The extraordinary in the ordinary: Skychology – an interpretative phenomenological analysis of looking up at the sky*, ResearchGate, March 2019.

4 S. Masoudinejad and T. Hartig, 'Window View to the Sky as a Restorative Resource for Residents in Densely Populated Cities', *Environment and Behavior*, 52(4), 2020, pp. 401–36.

5 B. Cresswell, diary, 9 June 1929, quoted in J. Burchardt, *Lifescapes: The Experience of Landscape in Britain 1870–1960*, Cambridge University Press, 2023.

6 A. Smalley, 'Beyond blue-sky thinking: Diurnal patterns and ephemeral meteorological phenomena impact appraisals of beauty, awe, and value in urban and natural landscapes', *Journal of Env. Psychology*, vol. 86, March 2023. Covered in 'Week 44: Seek out the Sublime' in my book, *52 Ways to Walk*.

7 Ibid.

8   M. van Elk, et al., 'The Neural Correlates of the Awe Experience: Reduced Default Mode Network Activity During Feelings of Awe', *Human Brain Mapping*, 7 May 2019, onlinelibrary.wiley.com/doi/full/10.1002/hbm.24616

9   M. D. Greicius, et al., 'Resting-state functional connectivity in major depression: abnormally increased contributions from subgenual cingulate cortex and thalamus', *Biol. Psychiatry*, 62(5), 1 September 2007, pp. 429–37. DOI: 10.1016/j.biopsych.2006.09.020

10 W. Gu, et al., 'Hyperactivity of the default-mode network in first-episode, drug-naive schizophrenia at rest revealed by family-based case-control and traditional case-control designs', *Medicine* (Baltimore), 96(13), March 2017, e6223. DOI: 10.1097/MD.0000000000006223

11 V. Okken, et al., 'When the World Is Closing In: Effects of Perceived Room Brightness and Communicated Threat During Patient-Physician Interaction', *HERD: Health Environments Research & Design Journal.*, 7(1), 2013, pp. 37–53. DIO: 10.1177/193758671300700104

12 V. Okken, et al., 'Room to Move: On Spatial Constraints and Self-Disclosure During Intimate Conversations', *Environment and Behavior*, 45(6), 2013, pp. 737–60.

13 T. J. L. van Rompay and T. Jol, 'Wild and Free: Unpredictability and Spaciousness as Predictors of Creative Performance', *Journal of Env. Psychology*, vol. 48, December 2016, www.sciencedirect.com/science/article/abs/pii/S0272494416300883?via%3Dihub NB: Creativity was self-reported from a very small sample size.

14 All quotes from G. Bachelard, *The Poetics of Space*, Penguin, 2014, p. 222.

15 S. Cao, et al., 'Cloudy or sunny? Effects of different environmental types of urban green spaces on public physiological and psychological health under two weather conditions', *Front. Public Health*, 11:1258848, 28 August 2023. DOI: 10.3389/fpubh.2023.1258848

9: CLIFFTOPS

1   D. Bair, *Simone de Beauvoir: A Biography*, Simon & Schuster, 1991, p. 174.

2   For a full account of de Beauvoir's walking, see either her memoir, *The Prime of Life*, or Chapter 6 of *Windswept: Why Women Walk* by A. Abbs, John Murray, 2021.

3   See for example: J. H. Park, et al., 'Sedentary Lifestyle: Overview of Updated Evidence of Potential Health Risks', *Korean J. Fam. Med.*, 41(6), November 2020, pp. 365–73. DOI: 10.4082/kjfm.20.0165

4 S. J. H. Biddle, et al., 'Device-assessed total and prolonged sitting time: associations with anxiety, depression, and health-related quality of life in adults', *J. Affect. Disord.*, 287, 15 May 2021, pp. 107–114. DOI: 10.1016/j.jad.2021.03.037

5 T. Huang, et al., 'Screen-based sedentary behaviors but not total sedentary time are associated with anxiety among college students', *Front. Public Health*, 10:994612, 20 October 2022. DOI: 10.3389/fpubh.2022.994612

6 E. Stamatakis, et al., 'Vigorous Intermittent Lifestyle Physical Activity and Cancer Incidence Among Nonexercising Adults: The UK Biobank Accelerometry Study', *JAMA Oncol.*, 9(9), 2023, pp. 1255–9. DOI:10.1001/jamaoncol.2023.1830

7 The Durham Heritage Coastal Path is a favourite walk of mine, featuring both the ruins of industry, the sea and cliffs, as is Spain's Lighthouse Way, with its blend of shoreline, hilltops and endless lighthouses.

10: LAKES

1 E. M. McGlashan, et al., 'Afraid of the dark: Light acutely suppresses activity in the human amygdala', *PLoS One*, 16(6), 16 June 2021, e0252350. DOI: 10.1371/journal.pone.0252350

2 I. Paparella, et al., 'Light modulates task-dependent thalamo-cortical connectivity during an auditory attentional task', *Commun. Biol.*, 6, 945, 2023. DOI: 10.1038/s42003-023-05337-5

3 K. Choi and H.-J. Suk, 'Dynamic lighting system for the learning environment: performance of elementary students', *Opt. Express*, 24, 2016, A907–A916.

4 A. C. Burns, et al., 'Day and night light exposure are associated with psychiatric disorders: an objective light study in > 85,000 people', *Nature Mental Health*, 2023. DOI: 10.1038/s44220023001358, www.nature.com/articles/s44220-023-00135-8. The biggest fall in risk was for self-harm and major depressive disorder.

5 D. C. Fernandez, et al., 'Light affects mood and learning through distinct retina–brain pathways', *Cell*, 175, 2018, pp. 71–84.e18.

6 C. W. McDougall, et al., 'Freshwater blue space and population health: An emerging research agenda,' *Sci. Total. Environ.*, 737:140196, 1 October 2016. DOI: 10.1016/j.scitotenv.2020.140196

7 J. E. Soler, et al., 'Daytime Light Intensity Modulates Spatial Learning and Hippocampal Plasticity in Female Nile Grass Rats (Arvicanthis niloticus)', *Neuroscience*, 404, 15 April 2019, pp. 175–83. DOI: 10.1016/j.neuroscience.2019.01.031

NOTES

8 A C. Burns, et al., 'Time spent in outdoor light is associated with mood, sleep, and circadian rhythm-related outcomes: A cross-sectional and longitudinal study in over 400,000 UK Biobank participants', *J. Affect. Disord.*, 295, 1 December 2021, pp. 347–52. DOI: 10.1016/j.jad.2021.08.056

9 Y. Mei, et al., 'Study on Emotional Perception of Hangzhou West Lake Scenic Area in Spring under the Influence of Meteorological Environment', *Int. J. Environ. Res. Public Health*, 20, 2023, 1905. DOI: 10.3390/ijerph20031905

10 M. Grace, et al., 'Using solicited research diaries to assess the restorative potential of exposure to inland blue space across time', *Landscape and Urban Planning*, vol. 241, 2024, 104904, ISSN 0169-2046. DOI: 10.1016/j.landurbplan.2023.104904

11 Communication with author, 27 October 2023.

12 C. Kelly, 'Ocean wellbeing-human wellbeing: blue space matters', Blue Planet Society, 7 December 2022, www.blueplanetsociety.org/ocean-wellbeing-human-wellbeing-blue-space-matters

13 Personal note to author, 27 October 2023.

14 H. Harati and T. Talhelm, 'Cultures in Water-Scarce Environments Are More Long-Term Oriented', *Psychol. Sci.*, 34(7), July 2023, pp. 754–70. DOI: 10.1177/09567976231172500

15 L. Luo, et al., 'Differentiating Mental Health Promotion Effects of Various Blue Spaces: An Electroencephalography Study', *Journal of Environmental Psychology*, vol. 88, June 2023. DOI: 10.1016/j.jenvp.2023.102010

16 S. Cao, et al., 'Cloudy or sunny? Effects of different environmental types of urban green spaces on public physiological and psychological health under two weather conditions', *Front. Public. Health.*, 11:1258848, 28 August 2023. DOI: 10.3389/fpubh.2023.1258848

17 D. K. Lynch and W. C. Livingston, *Colour and Light in Nature*, Cambridge University Press, 1995, p. 254.

18 Z. Zhang, et al., 'Self-Reported Outdoor Light Exposure Time and Incident Heart Failure', *J. Am. Heart Assoc.*, 13(4), 20 February 2024, e031830. DOI: 10.1161/JAHA.123. 031830

19 R. Parikh, et al., 'Seasonal AMH variability implies a positive effect of UV exposure on the deterioration of ovarian follicles', *Steroids*, 200:109307, December 2023. DOI: 10.1016/j.steroids.2023.109307

20 J. Shaw, 'Glittering Light on Water', *Optics and Photonics News*, vol. 10, issue 3, March 1999, pp. 43–5, 68.

11: GHOSTLANDS

1 Quoted in 'Walks on Old Railways Lines', *Heart Matters* (British Heart Foundation magazine), www.bhf.org.uk/informationsupport/heart-matters-magazine/activity/walking/railway-walks

2 E. Healey, 'The Lakenham Way', National Centre for Writing, 17 May 2019, nationalcentreforwriting.org.uk/writing-hub/read-the-lakenham-way-by-emma-healey

3 B. Korsten, 'Train Your Brain to be More Creative', *Harvard Business Review*, 17 June 2021, hbr.org/2021/06/train-your-brain-to-be-more-creative

4 P. Long, et al., 'Intranasal Oxytocin and Pain Reduction: Testing a Social Cognitive Mediation Model', *Brain Sci.*, 13(12), 7 December 2023, p. 1689. DOI: 10.3390/brainsci13121689

5 B. Buemann, 'Does activation of oxytocinergic reward circuits postpone the decline of the aging brain?', *Front. Psychol.*, 14, 29 December 2023, p. 1250745. DOI: 10.3389/fpsyg.2023.1250745

6 T. R. Jong, et al., 'Salivary oxytocin concentrations in response to running, sexual self-stimulation, breastfeeding and the TSST: The Regensburg Oxytocin Challenge (ROC) study', *Psychoneuroendocrinology*, 62, December 2015, pp. 381–8. DOI: 10.1016/j.psyneuen.2015.08.027

7 P. Grahn and K. Uvnäs-Moberg, 'The Oxytocinergic System as a Mediator of Anti-stress and Instorative Effects Induced by Nature: The Calm and Connection Theory', *Front. Psychol.*, 12, 5 July 2021, p. 617814. DOI: 10.3389/fpsyg.2021.617814

8 K. Murata, et al., 'Increase of tear volume in dogs after reunion with owners is mediated by oxytocin', *Current Biology*, vol. 32, issue 16, 22 August 2022, www.cell.com/current-biology/fulltext/S0960-9822(22)01132-0

9 'Why places matter to people', 2019 and 2017 National Trust/University of Surrey surveys, nt.global.ssl.fastly.net/binaries/content/assets/website/national/pdf/why-places-matter-to-people.pdf

10 J. A. Barraza and P. J. Zak, 'Empathy toward strangers triggers oxytocin release and subsequent generosity', *Ann N Y Acad. Sci.*, 1167, June 2009, pp. 182–9. DOI: 10.1111/j.1749-6632.2009.04504.x

11 T. M. Schladt, et al., 'Choir versus Solo Singing: Effects on Mood, and Salivary Oxytocin and Cortisol Concentrations', *Front. Hum. Neurosci.*, vol. 11, 14 September 2017, www.frontiersin.org/articles/10.3389/fnhum.2017.00430/full

12 G. Domes, et al., 'Oxytocin promotes facial emotion recognition and amygdala reactivity in adults with asperger syndrome', *Neuropsychopharmacology*, 39(3), February 2014, pp. 698–706. DOI: 10.1038/npp.2013.254

12: THERAPEUTIC LANDSCAPES

1 No cure has been recorded since 1976, at the time of writing.

2 B. François, et al., 'The Lourdes medical cures revisited', *J. Hist. Med. Allied. Sci.*, 69(1), January 2014, pp. 135–62. DOI: 10.1093/jhmas/jrs041

3 E. Rahtz, et al., 'Transcendent Experiences Among Pilgrims to Lourdes: A Qualitative Investigation', *J. Relig. Health.*, 60(6), December 2021, pp. 3788–806. DOI: 10.1007/s10943-021-01306-6

4 G. Perriam, 'Sacred Spaces, Healing Places: Therapeutic Landscapes of Spiritual Significance', *J. Med. Humanit.*, 36, 2015, pp. 19–33. DOI: 10.1007/s10912-014-9318-0

5 S. Yang, et al., 'Analysis of the Dong bao Ye as sacred landscape and its putative therapeutic mechanisms', *Health & Place*, vol. 83, 2023, 103102, ISSN 1353-8292. DOI: 10.1016/j.healthplace.2023.103102

6 'Aim 2', Stanford Mind & Body Lab, Research, mbl.stanford.edu/research

7 E. Sternberg, *Healing Spaces: The Science of Place and Well-Being*, Harvard University Press, 2009.

8 C. A. P. Faria, et al., 'Landscape and Senses in a Portuguese Municipality on the Way of St. James: Potential Impacts on the Well-Being of Pilgrims', *J. Relig. Health*, 4 August 2022, pp. 1–26. DOI: 10.1007/s10943-022-01617-2

9 S. L. Warber, et al., 'Healing the heart: a randomized pilot study of a spiritual retreat for depression in acute coronary syndrome patients', *Explore* (NY), 7(4), July–August 2011, pp. 222–33. DOI: 10.1016/j.explore.2011.04.002

10 G. Perriam, 'Sacred spaces, healing places: therapeutic landscapes of spiritual significance', *J. Med. Humanit.*, 36(1), March 2015, pp. 19–33. DOI: 10.1007/s10912-014-9318-0

11 C. Nolan, 'Sites of Existential Relatedness: findings from phenomenological research at Stonehenge, Avebury and the Vale of Pewsey, Wiltshire, UK', *Public Archaeology*, 18(1), 2019, pp. 28–51; C. Nolan. 'Prehistoric Landscapes as a Source of Ontological Security for the Present Day, Heritage & Society', 12:1, 2019, pp. 1–25, DOI: 10.1080/2159032X.2020.1818501; C. Nolan, 'Therapeutic Landscapes: Wellbeing and the Historic Environment', paper presented for the Athabasca Research Centre Webinar Series, 22 April 2021; Dr S. I. Dailoo, 'Therapeutic Landscapes: Wellbeing and the Historic Environment', https://www.youtube.com/watch?v=LqTyCeMTGoc

12 Author interview, 11 January 2024.

13 A. M. Globig, et al., 'The β_1-adrenergic receptor links sympathetic nerves to T cell exhaustion', *Nature*, 622, 2023, pp. 383–92. DOI: 10.1038/s41586-023-06568-6

14 In one study, participants who knew they were about to receive an electric shock were far less anxious than participants who were told they had a 50 per cent chance of receiving a shock (A. O. de Berker, R. B. Rutledge, et al., 'Computations of uncertainty mediate acute stress responses in humans', *Nature Communications*, 2016; 7: 10996. DOI: 10.1038/ncomms10996. We are wired to want certainty.

15 A. Lightman, *The Transcendent Brain: Spirituality in the Age of Science*, Pantheon, 2023.

16 J. Lindert, et al., 'Factors Contributing to Resilience Among First Generation Migrants, Refugees and Asylum Seekers: A Systematic Review', *Int. J. Public Health.*, 68:1606406, 11 December 2023. DOI: 10.3389/ijph.2023.1606406

17 H. Jafari, et al., 'The Association between Occupational Burnout and Spiritual Well-Being in Emergency Nurses: A Cross-Sectional Study', *Bull. Emerg. Trauma*, 11(4), 2023, pp. 184–9. DOI: 10.30476/BEAT.2023.98919.1444

18 M. Eglin, et al., 'Impact of social support and religiosity/spirituality on recovery from acute cardiac events and heart surgery in a Swiss study', *Int. J. Psychiatry Med.*, 29 December 2023, 912174231225801. DOI: 10.1177/00912174231225801

19 A. Barbieri and E. Rossero, '"It is like post-traumatic stress disorder, but in a positive sense!": New territories of the self as inner therapeutic landscapes for youth experiencing mental ill-health', *Health Place*, 85:103157, 3 December 2023. DOI: 10.1016/j.healthplace.2023.103157

20 See for example the work of A. Thorley and K. Petty, cited in *Wanderland: A Search for Magic in the Landscape* by J. Reddy (pp. 181 and 218), who describes 'thin places' as those 'where the walls between human, animal, element, matter and spirit are gossamer, and where highly charged encounters . . . are perfectly normal'.

21 E. Bendien, et al., 'A Dutch Study of Remarkable Recoveries After Prayer: How to Deal with Uncertainties of Explanation', *J. Relig. Health*, 62(3), June 2023, pp. 1731–55. DOI: 10.1007/s10943-023-01750-6

22 A. P. Stern, 'Hope: why it matters', Harvard Health Publishing, 16 July 2021, www.health.harvard.edu/blog/hope-why-it-matters-202107162547

13: CANAL TOWPATHS

1 R. McFarlane, 'These Are Our Waters', waterlines.org.uk/poems

2 M. Georgiou, et al., 'Mechanisms of Impact of Blue Spaces on Human Health: A Systematic Literature Review and Meta-Analysis', *Int. J. Environ. Res. Public Health*, 18(5), 2021, p. 2486; www.mdpi.com/1660-4601/18/5/2486

3 K. M. Heilman, 'Possible Brain Mechanisms of Creativity', *Arch. Clin. Neuropsychol.*, 31(4), June 2016, pp. 285–96. DOI: 10.1093/arclin/acw009

4 J. A. Easterbrook, 'The effect of emotion on cue utilization and the organization of behavior', *Psychological Review*, 66, 1959, pp. 180–201, pubmed.ncbi.nlm.nih.gov/13658305

5 A. D. Ekstrom, 'Cognitive Neuroscience: Why do we get lost when we are stressed', *Current Biology*, vol. 30, issue 10, 18 May 2020, pp. R439–R441, www.sciencedirect.com/science/article/pii/S0960982220304358. Author note: Never set off on a complicated, routeless walk if you're already feeling anxious and stressed!

6 Author interview, 18 March 2024.

7 X. Lu, et al., 'On Shape and the Computability of Emotions', *Proceedings of the 20th ACM International Conference on Multimedia*, Oct–Nov 2012, pp. 229–38. DOI: 10.1145/2393347. 2393384

8 E. K. Adam, et al., 'Diurnal cortisol slopes and mental and physical health outcomes: A systematic review and meta-analysis', *Psychoneuroendocrinology*, 83, September 2017, pp. 25–41. DOI: 10.1016/j.psyneuen.2017.05.018

9 C. Rominger, et al., 'Step-by-step to more creativity: The number of steps in everyday life is related to creative ideation performance', *Am. Psychol.*, 16 November 2023. DOI: 10.1037/amp0001232

10 Quoted in S. Pyrah, '"All it takes is a quick walk": how a few minutes' exercise can unleash creativity – even if you hate it', *The Guardian*, 4 March 2024, www.theguardian.com/lifeandstyle/2024/mar/04/all-it-takes-is-a-quick-walk-how-a-few-minutes-exercise-can-unleash-creativity-even-if-you-hate-it

11 'Why air pollution makes societies less creative', University of Cambridge Judge Business School, 19 January 2023, www.jbs.cam.ac.uk/insight/2023/why-air-pollution-makes-societies-less-creative

14: ECOTONES

1 E. Friedmann, et al., 'Companion animals and human health: Physical and cardiovascular influences', in *Companion Animals and Us: Exploring the Relationships between People and Pets*, Cambridge University Press, 2000, pp. 125–42.

2 R. E. Dick and J. C. Hendee, 'Human responses to encounters with wildlife in urban parks', *Leisure Sciences*, 8:1, 1986, pp. 63–77, DOI: 10.1080/01490408609513058

3 R. M. Yerbury and S. J. Luke, 'Human-Animal Interactions: Expressions of Wellbeing through a "Nature Language"', *Animals* (Basel), 11(4), 29 March 2021, p. 950. DOI: 10.3390/ani11040950

4 Ibid.

5 H. Macdonald, *Vesper Flights*, Jonathan Cape, 2020.

6 D. Cracknell, et al., 'Marine Biota and Psychological Well-Being: A Preliminary Examination of Dose-Response Effects in an Aquarium Setting', *Environ. Behav.*, 48(10), December 2016, pp. 1242–69. DOI: 10.1177/0013916515597512

7 R. Hammoud, et al., 'Smartphone-based ecological momentary assessment reveals mental health benefits of birdlife', *Sci. Rep.*, 12(1), 27 October 2022, p. 17589. DOI: 10.1038/s41598-022-20207-6

8 P. Zieris, et al., 'Nature experience and Wellbeing: Bird-watching as an Intervention in Nursing Homes to maintain cognitive resources, mobility and biopsychosocial health', *Journal of Environmental Psychology*, vol. 91, November 2023.

9 E. Stobbe, et al., 'Birdsongs alleviate anxiety and paranoia in healthy participants', *Sci. Rep.*, 12, 2022, 16414. DOI: 10.1038/s41598-022-20841-0

10 C. W. Butler, et al., 'Connection for conservation: The impact of counting butterflies on nature connectedness and wellbeing in citizen scientists', *Biological Conservation*, vol. 292, April 2024, www.sciencedirect.com/science/article/pii/S0006320724000582

11 J. Methorst, et al., 'The importance of species diversity for human well-being in Europe', *Ecological Economics*, vol. 181, March 2021. DOI: 10.1016/j.ecolecon.2020.106917

12 T. B. Smith, et al., 'Evolutionary consequences of human disturbance in a rainforest bird species from Central Africa', *Mol. Ecol.*, 17(1), January 2008, pp. 58–71. DOI: 10.1111/j.1365-294X.2007.03478.x

13 M. V. Lilly, et al., 'Eavesdropping grey squirrels infer safety from bird chatter', *PLOS ONE*, 14(9), 2014, e0221279. DOI: 10.1371/journal.pone.0221279

14 E. Ratcliffe, et al., 'Bird sounds and their contributions to perceived attention restoration and stress recovery', *Journal of Environmental Psychology*, vol. 36, 2013. DOI: 10.1016/j.jenvp.2013.08.004

15 A. J. Smalley, et al., 'Forest 404: Using a BBC drama series to explore the impact of nature's changing soundscapes on human wellbeing and behavior', *Glob. Environ. Change*, 74:102497, May 2022. DOI: 10.1016/j.gloenvcha.2022.102497

15: URBAN PARKS AND GARDENS

1 'Exposure to green spaces is key to preventing anxiety and depression in young people, study finds', UWE Bristol, 12 January 2021, www.uwe.ac.uk/news/exposure-to-green-spaces-is-key-to-preventing-anxiety-and-depression-in-young-people-study-finds

2 C. Song, et al., 'Physiological and Psychological Effects of a Walk in Urban Parks in Fall', *Int. J. Environ. Res. Public Health*, 12(11), 9 November 2015, pp. 14216–28. DOI: 10.3390/ijerph121114216

3 Q. Li, 'Effects of forest environment (Shinrin-yoku/Forest bathing) on health promotion and disease prevention – the Establishment of "Forest Medicine"', *Environmental Health and Preventive Medicine*, vol. 27, 2022, p. 43. DOI: 10.1265/ehpm.22-00160

4 L. Deng, et al., 'Empirical study of landscape types, landscape elements and landscape components of the urban park promoting physiological and psychological restoration', *Urban Forestry & Urban Greening*, vol. 48, February 2020, 126488.

5 For instance, Y. Zhai, et al., 'Seniors' Physical Activity in Neighborhood Parks and Park Design Characteristics', *Front. Public Health*, 8, July 2020, p. 322. DOI: 10.3389/fpubh.2020.00322

6 N. Kabisch, et al., 'Physiological and psychological effects of visits to different urban green and street environments in older people: A field experiment in a dense inner-city area', *Landscape and Urban Planning*, vol. 207, March 2021, www.sciencedirect.com/science/article/pii/S0169204620314821

7 L. Kong, et al., 'How do different types and landscape attributes of urban parks affect visitors' positive emotions?', *Landscape and Urban Planning*, October 2022 DOI: 10.1016/j.landurbplan.2022.104482

8 E. van Vliet, et al., 'The Influence of Urban Park Attributes on User Preferences: Evaluation of Virtual Parks in an Online Stated-Choice Experiment', *Int. J. Environ. Res. Public Health*, 18(1), 30 December 2020, p. 212. DOI: 10.3390/ijerph18010212

9 J. Martinez-Soto, et al., 'Exploring the Links Between Biophilic and Restorative Qualities of Exterior and Interior Spaces in Leon, Guanajuato, Mexico', *Front. Psychol.*, vol. 12, 17 August 2021, Sec. Environmental Psychology. DOI: 10.3389/fpsyg.2021.717116

16: OUTLANDS

1 C. Hickman, et al., 'Climate anxiety in children and young people and their beliefs about government responses to climate change: a global survey', *Lancet Planet Health*, 5(12), December 2021, e863–e873. DOI: 10.1016/S2542-5196(21)00278-3

2 T. Léger-Goodes, et al., 'Eco-anxiety in children: A scoping review of the mental health impacts of the awareness of climate change', *Front. Psychol.*, 13:872544, 25 July 2022. DOI: 10.3389/fpsyg.2022.872544

3 C. Rozuel and C. R. Bellehumeur, 'Contextualizing eco-anxiety and eco-anger: tentative responses to visceral and numinous emotions', *J. Anal. Psychol.*, 67(5), November 2022, pp. 1431–51. DOI: 10.1111/1468-5922.12870

4 J. Schomaker, 'Unexplored territory: Beneficial effects of novelty on memory', *Neurobiol. Learn. Mem.*, 161, May 2019, pp. 46–50. DOI: 10.1016/j.nlm.2019.03.005

5 Ibid.

6 N. Hunt, *Outlandish: Walking Europe's Unlikely Landscapes*, John Murray, 2021.

7 V. Breton-Provencher, et al., 'Spatiotemporal dynamics of noradrenaline during learned behaviour', *Nature*, 606, 2022, pp. 732–8 (2022). DOI: 10.1038/s41586-022-04782-2

8 K. Umejima, et al., 'Paper Notebooks vs. Mobile Devices: Brain Activation Differences During Memory Retrieval', *Front. Behav. Neurosci.*, 15:634158, 19 March 2021. DOI: 10.3389/fnbeh.2021.634158

17: DISTANCE TRAILS AND PILGRIM PATHS

1 M. Mau, et al., 'Mental movements: How long-distance walking influences reflection processes among middle-age and older adults', *Scandinavian Journal of Psychology*, 2021. DOI: 10.1111/sjop.12721

2 Csikszentmihalyi identified six common characteristics of the flow state: hyperfocused, task-specific attention; the merger of action and awareness, leading to total absorption in task engagement; the diminishment of self-reflective cognition and awareness of bodily processes; an altered perception of time; a heightened level of task performance accompanied by a feeling of complete control; and significant positive affect, including high levels of intrinsic reward, enjoyment, pleasure, euphoria and, often, increased feelings of meaning and purpose. Psychometrically, these six characteristics have become the way researchers both define and measure flow. Flow exists on a spectrum from the micro-flow, a low-intensity flow experience, to the macro-flow, a high-intensity flow experience.

3 Quotes from S. Kotler from his 2021 book *The Art of Impossible*.

4 S. Kotler, M. Mannino, et al., 'First few seconds for flow: A comprehensive proposal of the neurobiology and neurodynamics of state onset', *Neurosci. Biobehav. Rev.*, 143:104956, December 2022. DOI: 10.1016/j.neubiorev.2022.104956

NOTES

5   M. Kano, et al., 'Endocannabinoid-mediated control of synaptic transmission', *Physiol. Rev.*, 89 (1), 2009, pp. 309–80.

6   A. S. Mills and T. S. Butler, 'Flow Experience Among Appalachian Trail Thru-hikers', in J. G. Peden and R. M. Schuster (comps., eds.), *Proceedings of the 2005 northeastern recreation research symposium, 10–12 April 2005*, Bolton Landing, NY, 2006. Gen. Tech. Rep. NE-341. Newtown Square, PA: US Forest Service, Northeastern Research Station: 366–70.

7   M. Mau, et al., 'Are Long-Distance Walks Therapeutic? A Systematic Scoping Review of the Conceptualization of Long-Distance Walking and Its Relation to Mental Health', *Int. J. Environ. Res. Public Health*, 18(15), 21 July 2021, p. 7741. DOI: 10.3390/ijerph18157741

8   Flow may require some kind of stress response at the front end of the experience, according to Kotler, et al., 'First few seconds for flow . . .', 2022.

9   Author interview, 6 January 2024.

10 R. E. Saunders, et al., 'Personal transformation through long-distance walking', in *Tourist Experience and Fulfilment: Insights from positive psychology*, ed. S. Filep and P. Pearce, Routledge, 2014, pp.127–46.

11 Email correspondence with author, 9 October 2023.

12 Author interview by email, 10 October 2023.

13 Author interview, 15 June 2024. See also P. van Lange and S. Columbus, 'Vitamin S: Why is Social Contact, Even With Strangers, So Important to Well-Being?', *Current Directions in Psychological Science*, vol. 30, issue 3, 27 May 2021. DOI: 10.1177/09637214211002538

14 J. Fuss, et al., 'A runner's high depends on cannabinoid receptors in mice', *Proc. Natl Acad. Sci. USA*, 112(42), 20 October 2015, pp. 13105–8. DOI: 10.1073/pnas.1514996112

15 D. Mitten, et al., 'Hiking: A Low-Cost, Accessible Intervention to Promote Health Benefits', *Am. J. Lifestyle Med.*, 12(4), 9 July 2016, pp. 302–10. DOI: 10.1177/1559827616658229

16 S. Anzman-Frasca, et al., 'Effects of a randomized controlled hiking intervention on daily activities, sleep, and stress among adults during the COVID-19 pandemic', *BMC Public Health*, 23(1), 15 May 2023, p. 892. DOI: 10.1186/s12889-023-15696-7

17 For more on the mind-blowing benefits of walking in a group, see A. Abbs, *52 Ways to Walk*, 'Week 43: Walk with Others'.

18 K. Redick, 'Spiritual rambling: long distance wilderness sojourning as meaning-making', *Journal of Ritual Studies*, vol. 30, 2016, www.academia.edu/37171546/Spiritual_Rambling_Long_Distance_Wilderness_Sojourning_as_Meaning_Making

19 S. Tykarski and F. Mróz, 'The Pilgrimage on the Camino de Santiago and Its Impacts on Marital and Familial Relationships: An Exploratory Study', *J. Relig. Health*, 1 May 2023, pp. 1–24. DOI: 10.1007/s10943-023-01825-4

20 V. Lange and Columbus, 'Vitamin S'.

21 D. Rosen, et al., 'Creative flow as optimized processing: Evidence from brain oscillations during jazz improvisations by expert and non-expert musicians', *Neuropsychologia*, 196, 2024, p. 108824. DOI: 10.1016/j.neuropsychologia.2024.108824

18: MOUNTAINS

1 Quoted in ncert.nic.in/textbook/pdf/hehd105.pdf

2 All quotes from N. Shepherd, *The Living Mountain*, written 1944, published 1977.

3 J. Wapner, interview with *Scientific American*: 'Vision and Breathing May Be the Secrets to Surviving 2020', 16 November 2020, www.scientificamerican.com/article/vision-and-breathing-may-be-the-secrets-to-surviving-2020

4 For more on this see Week 8, 'Walk with Vista Vision' in *52 Ways to Walk*.

5 F. Pessoa, *The Book of Disquiet*, 1982.

6 E. Kim, et al., 'Is altitude a determinant of the health benefits of nature exposure? A systematic review and meta-analysis', *Front. Public Health*, 25 November 2022, www.frontiersin.org/articles/10.3389/fpubh.2022.1021618/full

7 K. Miskowiak, et al., 'Erythropoietin improves mood and modulates the cognitive and neural processing of emotion 3 days post administration', *Neuropsychopharmacology*, 33(3), February 2008, pp. 611–8. DOI: 10.1038/sj.npp.1301439

8 The human brain is the most complex object in the known universe. It is the most fascinating and the most mysterious. The entire variety of human experience, all our emotions, our perceptions, our sensations are housed in those 1,300 grams of interconnected tissue. See also interview in C. Southwick, 'We Know Exercise Prevents Cancer. A New Study Tells Us Why', *Medscape*, 4 October 2023, www.medscape.com/s/viewarticle/997091?src=rss&form=fpf

9 J. Álvarez-Herms and A. Odriozola, 'Microbiome and physical activity', *Adv. Genet.*, 111, 2024, pp. 409–50. DOI: 10.1016/bs.adgen.2024.01.002

10 D. Liu, et al., 'Moderate altitude exposure impacts host fasting blood glucose and serum metabolome by regulation of the intestinal flora', *Sci. Total Environ.*, 905, 20 December 2023, p. 167016. DOI: 10.1016/j.scitotenv.2023.167016

11 A. Arnberger, et al., 'Health-Related Effects of Short Stays at Mountain Meadows, a River and an Urban Site – Results from a Field Experiment', *Int. J. Environ. Res. Public Health*, 15, 2018, p. 2647. DOI: 10.3390/ijerph15122647

12 R.-L. Ghe, et al., 'Determinants of erythropoietin release in response to short-term hypobaric hypoxia', *Journal of Applied Physiology*, 1 June 2002, DOI: 10.1152/japplphysiol. 00684.2001

13 A. Arnberger, et al., 'Health-Related Effects . . .'.

19: RIVERS

1 E. C. Meyer, et al., 'Predictors of recovery from post-deployment posttraumatic stress disorder symptoms in war veterans: The contributions of psychological flexibility, mindfulness, and self-compassion', *Behav. Res. Ther.*, 114, March 2019, pp. 7–14. DOI: 10.1016/j.brat.2019.01.002

2 E. Britton, et al., 'Blue care: a systematic review of blue space interventions for health and wellbeing', *Health Promot. Int.*, 35(1), 1 February 2020, pp. 50–69. DOI: 10.1093/heapro/ day103

3 N. Bergou, et al., 'The mental health benefits of visiting canals and rivers: An ecological momentary assessment study', *PLoS One*, 17(8), 31 August 2022, e0271306. DOI: 10.1371/ journal.pone.0271306

4 A. Arnberger, et al., 'Health-Related Effects of Short Stays at Mountain Meadows, a River and an Urban Site – Results from a Field Experiment', *Int. J. Environ. Res. Public Health*, 15, 2018, p. 2647. DOI: 10.3390/ijerph15122647

5 E. Frohmann, et al., 'Psychologische Effekte atmosphärischer Qualitäten der Landschaft', *Schweiz. Z. Forstwes.*, 161, 2010, pp. 97–103.

6 Negative air ions have been found to improve respiration, immunity and inflammation among adults, children and Covid-19 patients. More information can be found in Week 30 of my book, *52 Ways to Walk*, Bloomsbury, 2022.

7 Quoted in W. Nichols, *Blue Mind: How water makes you happier, more connected and better at what you do*, Abacus, 2018, p. 89.

8 T. Börger, et al., 'The value of blue-space recreation and perceived water quality across Europe: A contingent behaviour study', *Sci. Total Environ.*, 771, 1 June 2021, 145597. DOI: 10.1016/j.scitotenv.2021.145597

9 K. Hu, et al., 'Modifying temperature-related cardiovascular mortality through green-blue space exposure', *Environ. Sci. Ecotechnol.*, 20, 7 March 2024, 100408. DOI: 10.1016/j.ese.2024.100408

10 V. Vitale, et al., 'Mechanisms underlying childhood exposure to blue spaces and adult subjective wellbeing', *Journal of Environmental Psychology*, vol. 84, December 2022, DOI: 10.1016/j.jenvp.2022.101876

11 L. Luo, et al., 'Differentiating Mental Health Promotion Effects of Various Blue Spaces: An Electroencephalography Study', *Journal of Environmental Psychology*, vol. 88, June 2023, DOI: 10.1016/j.jenvp.2023.102010

20: NOCTURNE

1 From 'Lecture to her pupils at Vassar', 1865.

2 Quotes sourced from *My Faraway One: Selected Letters of Georgia O'Keeffe and Alfred Stieglitz, vol. 1 1915–1933*, ed. S. Greenough, 2011.

3 A. Abbs, *Windswept: Why Women Walk*, Two Roads, 2021.

4 For more, see A. Abbs, *Sleepless: Discovering the Power of the Night Self*, John Murray, 2024.

5 C. Grillon, et al., 'Darkness facilitates the acoustic startle reflex in humans', *Biol. Psychiatry*, 42(6), 15 September 1997, pp. 453–60. DOI: 10.1016/S0006-3223(96)00466-0

6 A. Caruso, et al., 'Corticotropin-Releasing Hormone: Biology and Therapeutic Opportunities', *Biology*, 11, 2022, 1785. DOI: 10.3390/biology11121785

7 'Corticotrophin-releasing hormone', You and your hormones, www.yourhormones.info/hormones/corticotrophin-releasing-hormone

8 F. Williams, 'Awe Is Good for Your Brain. Here's How to Find It', *Outside*, 25 July 2023, www.outsideonline.com/adventure-travel/essays/power-of-awe

9 A. C. Burns, et al., 'Day and night light exposure are associated with psychiatric disorders: an objective light study in >85,000 people', *Nat. Mental Health*, 1, 2023, pp. 853–62. DOI: 10.1038/s44220-023-00135-8, and follow-up interview with author, 16 November 2023.

10 B. Barbini, et al., 'Dark therapy for mania: a pilot study', *Bipolar Disord.*, 7, 2005, pp. 98–101. DOI: 10.1111/j.1399-5618.2004.00166.x

11 C. Barnes, 'Development and testing of the Night Sky Connectedness Index (NSCI)', *Journal of Environmental Psychology*, vol. 93, January 2024. DOI: 10.1016/j.jenvp.2023.102198

12 Author interview, December 2023.

13 S. Takeuchi, et al., 'The circadian clock in the piriform cortex intrinsically tunes daily changes of odor-evoked neural activity', *Commun. Biol.*, 6, 2023, p. 332. DOI: 10.1038/s42003-023-04691-8

14 Author interview, January 2024.

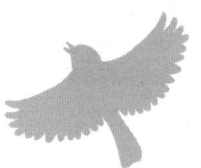

Index

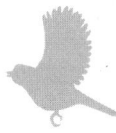

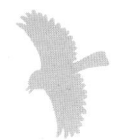

INDEX

A Note on the Author

———————

Annabel Streets is an award-winning writer of eight books. As Annabel Streets, she is the author of the international bestseller, *52 Ways to Walk*. As Annabel Abbs, she is the author of *Windswept: Why Women Walk*, a 2021 top 10 travel book, and the international bestseller, *The Language of Food*. Her work has been translated into over 30 languages. Annabel writes for a wide range of publications, is a fellow of the Brown Foundation, and lives in London and Sussex. She can be found on foot and at @annabelabbs.

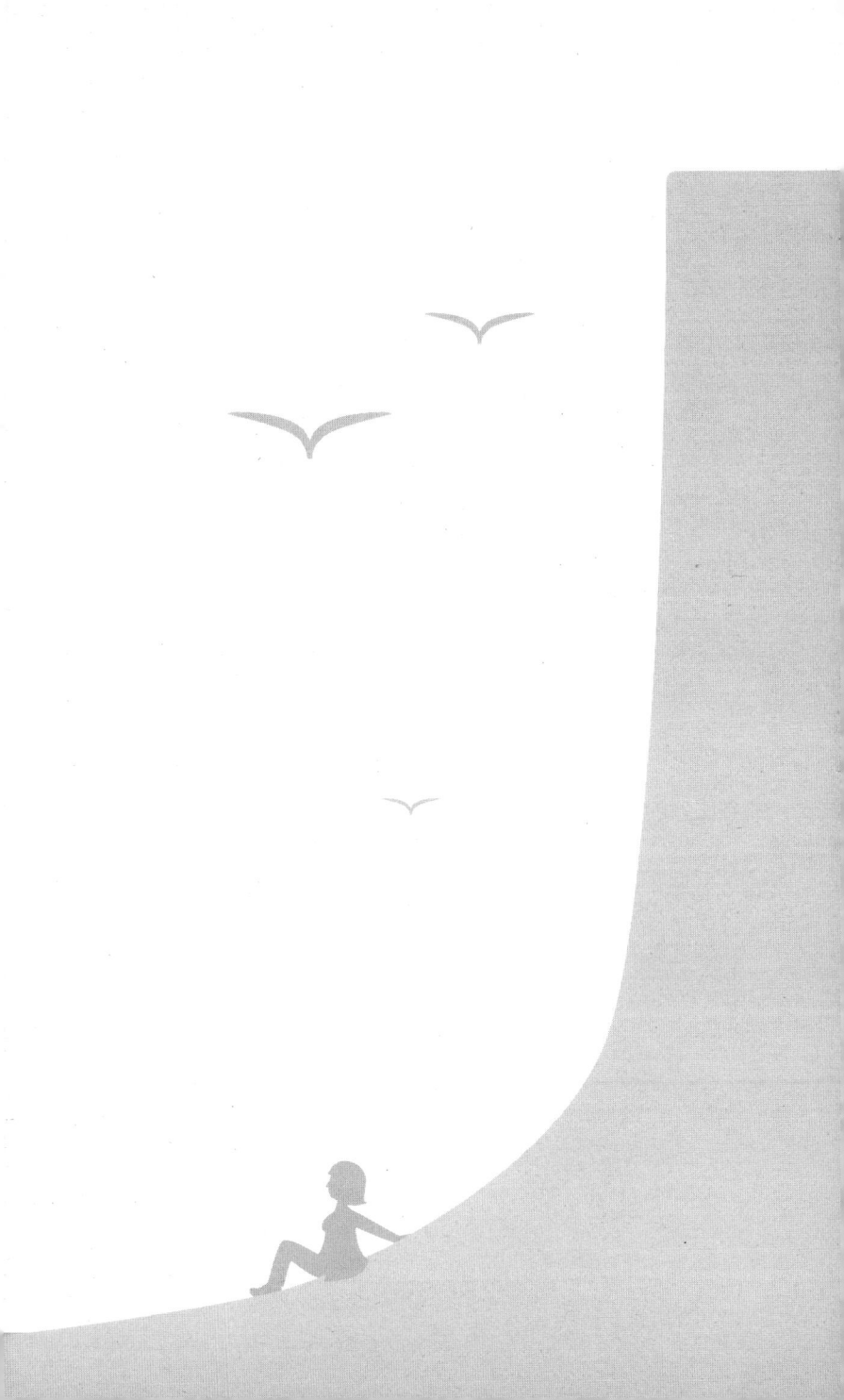

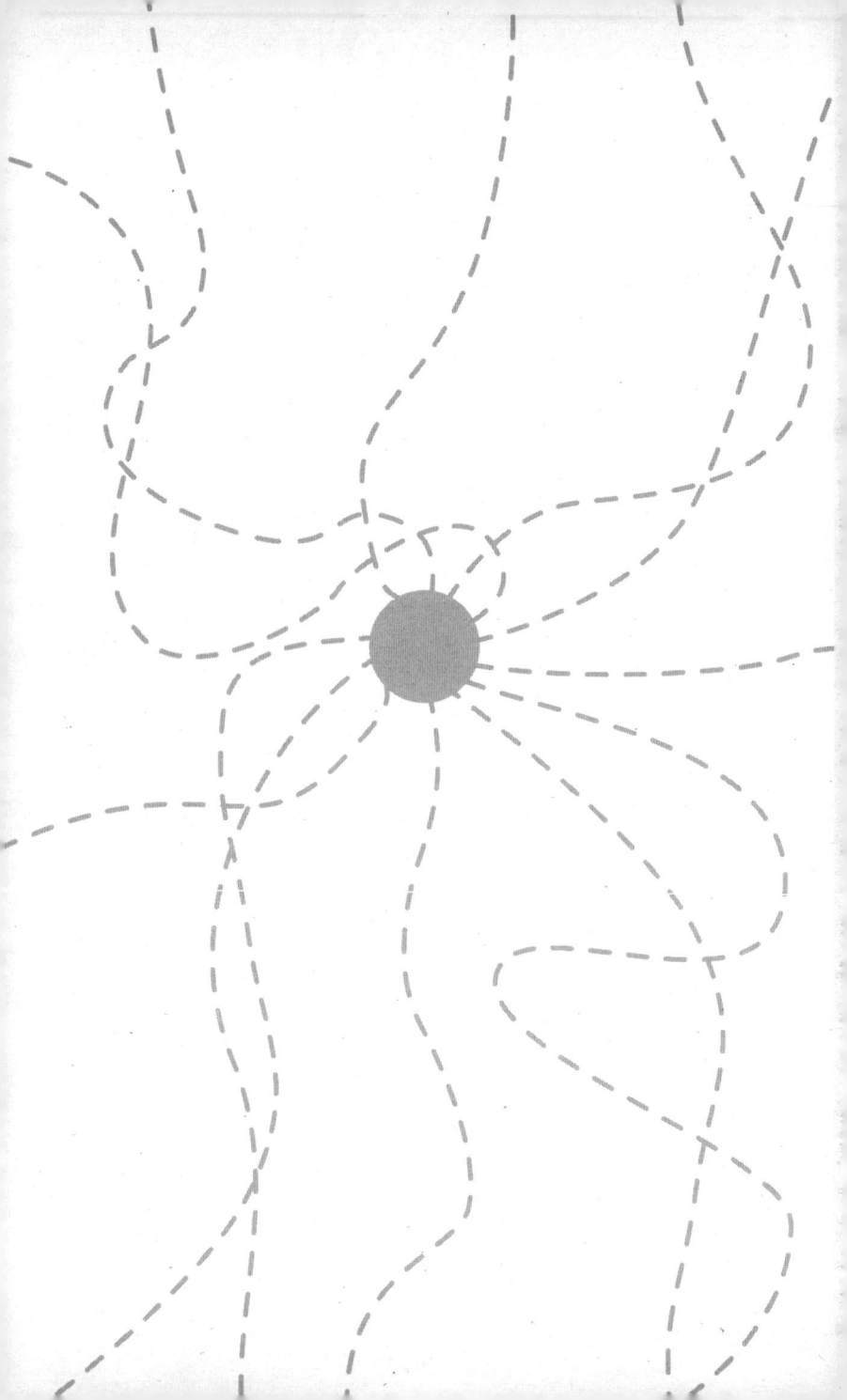